LOSING CLIVE
TO YOUNGER
ONSET DEMENTIA

of related interest

Dancing with Dementia
My Story of Living Positively with Dementia
Christine Bryden
ISBN 978 1 84310 332 5
eISBN 978 1 84642 095 5

Who will I be when I die?
Christine Bryden
ISBN 978 1 84905 312 9
eISBN 978 0 85700 645 5

Dementia - Support for Family and Friends
Dave Pulsford and Rachel Thompson
ISBN 978 1 84905 243 6
eISBN 978 0 85700 504 5

The Simplicity of Dementia
A Guide for Family and Carers
Huub Buijssen
ISBN 978 1 84310 321 9
eISBN 978 1 84642 096 2

Can I tell you about Dementia?
A guide for family, friends and carers
Jude Welton
ISBN 978 1 84905 297 9
eISBN 978 0 85700 634 9

Telling Tales About Dementia
Experiences of Caring
Edited by Lucy Whitman
ISBN 978 1 84310 941 9
eISBN 978 0 85700 017 0

A Personal Guide to Living with Progressive Memory Loss
Sandy Burgener and Prudence Twigg
ISBN 978 1 84310 863 4
eISBN 978 1 84642 719 0

Hearing the Person with Dementia
Person-Centred Approaches to Communication for Families and Caregivers
Bernie McCarthy
ISBN 978 1 84905 186 6
eISBN 978 0 85700 499 4

LOSING CLIVE
TO YOUNGER
ONSET DEMENTIA

HELEN BEAUMONT

*Foreword by Robin Jacoby, Professor Emeritus of
Old Age Psychiatry, The University of Oxford*

Jessica Kingsley *Publishers*
London and Philadelphia

First published in 2009
by Jessica Kingsley Publishers
73 Collier Street
London N1 9BE, UK
and
400 Market Street, Suite 400
Philadelphia, PA 19106, USA

www.jkp.com

Library of Congress Cataloging in Publication Data
Beaumont, Helen.
  Losing Clive to younger onset dementia : one family's story / Helen Beaumont.
    p. cm.
    ISBN 978-1-84310-480-3 (pb : alk. paper) 1. Beaumont, Clive--Mental health. 2. Presenile dementia--Patients--Great Britain--Biography. I. Title.
    RC522.B43 2009
    362.196'830092--dc22
                                                            2008025701

British Library Cataloguing in Publication Data
A CIP catalogue record for this book is available from the British Library

ISBN 978 1 84310 480 3
eISBN 978 1 84642 862 3

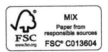

To Dave,
who gave me a reason to write this,

and to Dawn,
who helped me to keep going.

Contents

Foreword

One morning in the second half of the 1990s I received a phone call from a woman who was demanding to know why her husband was not permitted to wear a radio tracking device. Together with some colleagues in the University, I was running some experimental trials on the ethics and practicalities of tracking devices in patients suffering from dementia. The company who had loaned us the apparatus, which they had developed to track animals in the wild, had informed me that they were not prepared to take the legal risk of letting it be used in a patient with a cardiac pacemaker. They had admitted to me that there was no theoretical reason why their device should interfere with a pacemaker, but they did not want to take the risk of being sued.

I explained this to the woman who rang me, but she was having none of it. She told me that she was a physicist by training and had some understanding of the technology. Furthermore, she was perfectly capable of weighing up the risks involved and had judged them (quite correctly, as it happens) to be negligible. She was prepared to sign a document saying that she would not sue the company, although she did not conceal her contempt for its defensive attitude. She was determined to have the tracking device for her husband, and have it she did.

This was my first encounter with Helen Beaumont, which I should sum up as one in which a reasonable but iron determination prevailed. Although I did not personally have any responsibility for her husband's care, I knew about him because I was clinical director of the OPTIMA project, a dementia research study in Oxford, and Clive was a participant. This book is the story of him, his illness, his death and the legacy that Helen has made for him with The Clive Project.

When I was a medical student at a famous London teaching hospital, dementia was occasionally regarded by the medical profession as interesting but most often as a nuisance. Early onset cases were interesting because they were rare, but once the diagnosis had been made the patients were more or less told to go away and lump it. The majority of patients with dementia in those days, as now, were elderly, and doctors regarded them as a nuisance to be removed as soon as possible from an acute hospital bed to a long-stay ward at the back of a local mental hospital. It was not until the 1970s that pathologists and other medical scientists came to the conclusion that there was no difference pathologically between the rare early onset and common late onset cases. It was in this decade that science and the medical profession began to take dementia seriously and not simply regard it as a nuisance.

What exactly is dementia and how does it differ from Alzheimer's disease? Dementia is a syndrome, that is to say a collection of signs and symptoms diagnosed in life, which can be caused by a wide variety of underlying disease processes. Broadly speaking, the signs and symptoms are a global impairment of brain function that can include memory, language, motor and social skills, judgment and many other functions. In the majority of cases, but not all, deterioration is gradual and progressive. The commonest underlying disease causing dementia in western society is Alzheimer's disease, but there are many other causes – well over 50 in fact. Most of these are exceedingly rare.

In recent years much more attention has been paid to improving the management of dementia, especially the humane and ethical aspects of care. A small sign of this has been the abandonment of the terms 'pre-senile' and 'senile' with their negative connotations in favour of early- and late-onset. Society as a whole is far less tolerant of peremptory dismissal of dementia sufferers by doctors, although the Beaumonts' experience of the first neurologist who saw Clive is more typical of what happened when I was a medical student. The emergence of the Alzheimer's Society has been a powerful force for the change of attitude among lay people and professionals alike, whilst high-profile cases in the media, such as Iris Murdoch and Ronald Reagan, have increased general awareness of dementia.

Nevertheless, the special difficulties occasioned by early onset dementia, and the lack of services for them, remain a largely unsolved problem. Helen Beaumont's story of Clive brings this home in the most acute and moving way. Nowadays, when an older person's behaviour or memory changes, many people are alert to the possibility of a dementing process. In a younger person, as shown by Clive's story, disturbance and impairment can be quite advanced and noticeable to all before the penny drops that illness might be the cause. In my professional life I have seen this all too often.

Dementia in middle age brings special problems not usually associated with dementia in old age: coping with young children in the same home; coping with an employer who thinks you're incompetent, not sick; coping with the loss of income when the savings safety-net is not fully formed; and a host of other difficulties, many of which Helen Beaumont describes in this book.

To the outsider with no experience of dementia the mere thought of it induces a shudder, and the imagined prospect of it is one of unalloyed gloom. From my perspective as a professional, but nonetheless an outsider, those who are determined to make something positive out of the experience are also in some way ennobled and enriched by it, although I hasten to add that I definitely do not believe that suffering is necessarily ennobling or enriching. Who can doubt, however, that the creation of the The Clive Project, a service for early onset dementia sufferers where none existed before, has been one of the most positive outcomes of this story. I know of at least one other NHS service in a large English city that was set up and modelled on The Clive Project.

As far as Clive and Helen, themselves, are concerned, I found their story instructive, sobering, sometimes funny, and certainly moving. On occasions it made me angry at the behaviour of us professionals, but I learnt a great deal from it and I am certain that others will have the same experience as I have in reading this memorable book.

Robin Jacoby
Professor Emeritus of Old Age Psychiatry
The University of Oxford

Chapter 1

Beginnings

It's a Saturday morning in 1993. We're all in the living room, and the rain is beating against the window. Clive is sitting on the floor poring over the jobs section of the local paper; I am on the sofa with Alan on my knee; Rachel is playing quietly in a corner. It has become one of the many rituals that I dread. We are looking through the paper for jobs for Clive to apply for. I am irritated because I want to be doing the host of chores that is waiting for me. Clive is out of work, so I can't see why he can't do these himself and instead leaves them for me to do in my precious free time. I am also irritated because I can't see why we have to look at the paper together. Why can't he do this himself? However, it has become a routine, and it is very important for all of us that Clive get a job, so I try to hide my irritation, and concentrate on the paper. Teachers? No – not Clive. No qualifications (Oxford biochemistry degree apparently doesn't count). Drivers? No HGV or PSV licence. Clive turns the page, and looks interested and enthusiastic. I lean over his shoulder and look. Christ Church College is looking for porters and security men. That sounds good to Clive. I look at the salary offered, and then point out that the wages they offer are what we would have to pay a childminder, and so we would in fact be worse off if he took that job. I ask acidly why a recently retired Army Major, with said Oxford degree, and experience in bomb disposal and ammunition movement and storage, should want a job directing tourists round Christ Church – surely his ambitions run higher than that. Clive gives me a long, despairing look and turns the page.

It's one of the great regrets of my life that I let that opportunity slip by. I can understand now, knowing what I know now, why Clive couldn't and didn't explain to me why he was keen to apply for a job as college porter. He had never been one to explain himself to others, being a believer in the 'least said, soonest mended' school of thought. He was already having increasing difficulty with language – a symptom of the illness no-one yet knew he had. But I was the eloquent, articulate one, good with words, good at understanding things; the one who believed in sorting things out, the one who was not ill. The truth is that by then I was sick of trying to 'sort things out' with Clive. We could have conversations and apparently come to decisions which he later ignored. It never occurred to me that he had an illness which was slowly destroying his abilities to read, to talk, to comprehend the world about him. It was a realisation that came slowly over the next months and years. But I still regret losing that moment.

So where did it start, this illness that stole Clive away from us before we realised that anything was wrong? It's a very difficult question, and one with no clear answer. My best guess is in the late 1980s. We had returned from Dubai, where we had been living for a few years. For complicated reasons I stayed longer than Clive, but we were together again from May 1986. It felt great to be back together – we bought a house, and I started haunting DIY shops.

I was very much enjoying doing up the house. The people we bought from had been very heavy smokers, and it all needed redecorating – new bathroom, new kitchen, new carpets and curtains –all great fun for me, but not really Clive's cup of tea, and I was wondering what we could do together. I came up with what seemed to me to be a brilliant idea – I would learn to fly.

Clive had learnt to fly very soon after we were married, paying for the lessons with an inheritance from his grandad. After that, everywhere we went Clive found the local flying club and kept in a few hours a month. He had really wanted to join the RAF like his father, but his eyesight wasn't good enough to be a pilot. It seemed quite a good thing for me to learn – Clive could help me with the theory, and then we could maybe buy a share in a plane and go gadding off at weekends. Clive was very unenthusiastic when I suggested it to him, and a little later announced that he had decided to give up flying. What he said was that he couldn't afford to do enough hours to be safe. He wasn't prepared to discuss it any further, and so I just accepted his decision. Was this an early symptom of his illness, or just an unrelated incident? I wish we had been able to talk about it more, but at the time there were other things on our minds.

Clive had become more and more insistent that he wanted a family. This was another of the many things we never discussed when we married – Clive probably assumed family would come along, and I always thought that I was not the maternal type. I never had much strong maternal instinct; when my sister-in-law proudly gave me her new daughter to hold, I was very scared that I would hurt such a small, fragile bundle. I had a job (well, as Clive moved a lot, a succession of jobs) which I enjoyed, hobbies and friends, and plans for the future which I didn't want to give up. It was all very well for Clive to talk about starting a family – there was no expectation that he would give up his job to stay home and look after the children. And, of course, it was me that would have to be pregnant, and even the most well-intentioned book or friend admitted that giving birth was hard work. So Clive had to talk very long and hard to get me to agree. He could be very persuasive, and I felt fairly secure that he wouldn't leave me in the lurch, so I agreed. I did make a proviso that I would stay put with the family. I had enjoyed moving around the world with Clive, but I didn't think it would be the same with small children to care for. Most places we went I spent the first few weeks driving round quite lost, trying to find my way to the shops, the bank, the sports centre, and even my way home. I couldn't see that being quite so much of an adventure with children in the back of the car.

While I was pregnant, we discussed the last holiday we would have on our own, and agreed to go cycling in France. I bought a bike (Clive already had one, and used it to cycle the 12 miles to work and back), and we had a couple of gentle Sunday afternoon bike rides. After one of these, Clive came back with tickets for a holiday in Tenerife. It was a very good holiday, and I assumed he had decided my cycling was too gentle for him and didn't want to hurt my feelings.

Rachel was born in March 1988. Clive adored her. He hated to be away more than was necessary, and was driving back one evening from an exercise in the Thames Estuary when he crashed the car into the lane divider on the motorway. Fortunately no other car was involved, and his was still driveable. He made no fuss – Clive never did – but got back into the rather battered car, finished the drive home, told no-one but me and quietly got the car repaired. He assumed he had fallen asleep at the wheel. Maybe he did. Maybe the accident had nothing to do with what was to come. But it was the first accident he had had in 20 years.

A few weeks later he noticed an irregularity in his heartbeat. It was not causing him any drama, but he always got things checked out. The GP he was with then referred him to the Oxford hospital, who fitted him with a 24-hour monitoring tape. I delivered the tape to the hospital, and Clive went off for another Army job. It was Friday. Just after I returned home from dropping the tape, the telephone rang. It was the hospital. Could Clive come in immediately for a check-up? I explained he was away, and we agreed that he could come in on Monday, when he would be back. 'Oh', they said 'and don't worry, there really isn't a problem, but it would be better if he didn't drive too much before then'. I visualised Clive driving back to Oxford from the Isle of Man, and said that was OK. My imagination went into overdrive. Rachel was four months old. I was feeling particularly seedy and sorry for myself with undiagnosed early-morning sickness, and Clive was away. He had not informed the Army about what was going on – not something I was happy about, but he was adamant. He was back on Sunday, took a few days leave, and turned up at the hospital on Monday morning. I went with him. I can't remember who looked after Rachel – it is possible I took her with us as she was still very small and portable, but it was also a time when we did normal things like finding babysitters to leave children with.

A few hours later we were told Clive had sino-atrial disease, which is a problem with the heart's natural pacemaker. It's common in the elderly, but almost unheard of in an otherwise extremely fit middle-aged man. However, the consultant was very clear. This was what was wrong with Clive – the palpitations he had been having were only the start of what could be a very serious problem. The solution was fairly simple – fit a pacemaker – and his only concern was what was the best sort of pacemaker. They could fit a modern pacemaker that would allow Clive to continue his active lifestyle – running marathons, scuba diving, jumping out of aeroplanes… He would have to be careful going through airport security checks, but otherwise he could continue life as normal. So this was what he proposed to do.

Was the heart problem connected with his subsequent illness? I don't know. There is no known link between dementia and sino-atrial disease, but it seems to me very strange that something should stop the control centre of Clive's heart working properly a few years before he developed a disease of the brain – the body's control centre.

Clive and I needed to talk. I was not happy myself. I could not imagine the Army would be happy to let Clive continue in his current job with a heart problem, however benign. Clive liked his job, and wanted to keep it. He decided to have the pacemaker fitted, and tell no-one. He would not be talked out of it. The heart specialists knew what his job entailed, and were happy that it would be safe to continue with a pacemaker, and not safe to continue without. The pacemaker was fitted. All my worries seemed to be groundless. Life continued, fairly happily, for a while. Alan was born in March 1989. After a few months, I found myself a part-time job.

There were a few disagreements, but I could easily convince myself they were normal. After several months, Clive couldn't remember the names of the people I worked with. He had a curious blind spot about remembering when I had arranged to go out and he was expected to babysit. He always used to be an avid reader, and I noticed that he had stopped reading books. But then, I hardly read too many books myself those days. Clive loved the children, and was a very modern, hands-on dad. We were a very happy family practically all the time.

I got really annoyed with Clive when he decided to adopt a friend's cat – the friend was posted to Germany and couldn't take the cat without considerable expense. I was quite happy to have the cat, but Clive asked me when Alan was only about a month old, and I was still struggling to cope with two babies. I said I was happy to have the cat, but please not until the day before Clive's friend left for Germany. Clive agreed that seemed reasonable, and then came home that evening with the cat in a basket. No cat food. No litter tray. Just the cat, which he decanted from the basket. Then he went out for the evening. I was not happy.

A few weeks later we were due to go on holiday. I wanted to go diving in the Isle of Wight; Clive wanted to visit some friends in the Isle of Man. Instead of deciding which was possible in the ten days we had off, Clive decided we could do both. We would drive 250 miles to his mother's house, leave the children there, drive another 100 miles to the Isle of Man, spend three days there with his friends, return to pick the children up, drive to the Isle of Wight, set up camp there and I could go diving. I knew who would be organising the camping, the ferry tickets, the packing, the children… Clive would not be persuaded that the plan was impractical; I was too pig-headed to give up my diving. Eventually I invented a crisis at work that meant I couldn't get any time off at all, and we stayed home.

We had more holiday trouble at Christmas. I wanted to visit some good friends in Dubai, and Clive somewhat unwillingly agreed to come as well. I booked tickets, and eventually set about getting ready to go. We were flying from Gatwick, and parking at the airport. The journey normally took two hours, so I thought leaving three hours before we needed to be there would be plenty. Clive disagreed, but didn't tell me until half an hour before he wanted to leave, when he started agitating about being late. Getting ready was not trivial, as we were travelling with two toddlers, and I wanted to leave the house in some sort of order. Things got more and more heated, until Clive went off in a huff and sat in the car, blowing the horn and revving the engine from time to time. This is a story many parents will recognise, and only worth noting because it showed a side of Clive I had never seen before in the almost 20 years I had known him. Clive had been selected by the Army for training in bomb disposal. They don't select men who are excitable or have a bad temper. Clive had always been imperturbable – bomb-proof, indeed. I got my act together as quickly as possible, and we set off to the airport. Most unusually, I was driving. As we drove down the M25, Clive demanded that I stop the car immediately, as he wanted to get out – he had decided against coming. He didn't want driving to the nearest town, or even the next exit; he wanted to be left on the hard shoulder. I managed to jolly him along, and we got to the airport, and eventually out to Dubai, where Clive declared he had flu, and took to his bed for a few days. He certainly wasn't well – this was a man who never had colds or flu.

When we came home, things settled down again for a few months, and were pretty much OK until Clive came home from work with, as he put it, 'a proposition he would like to put to me'. How would it be if we all moved down to Salisbury?

He was due a posting (the Army moves its people around quite regularly), and had been steadfastly refusing all attempts to post him to a desk job in London. Clive was never one for desk jobs if they could be avoided. He was also getting somewhat depressed about not getting promoted, and I could never persuade him that maybe the two might go together. The possibility of a job had come up near Salisbury. It was a job for which he was very well qualified, and might give him the promotion if he did well, but…it was in Salisbury, and that was too far to travel daily. He wanted his family with him; there was a house there; would I move?

This was breaking the agreement we had made when we started the family: that we would buy a house and settle down. I never fancied the idea of moving around every two years with children in tow. It was fine when there were just the two of us, but this was different. Still, Clive really wanted the job, and the children had not yet started playschool, so there wouldn't be too much disruption for them. It would mean losing my job, but I had always managed to find something. So on the whole I could find no cogent reason for refusing. I'm ashamed to say it put me in a bad mood for a very long time. I should have refused, or agreed and gone along wholeheartedly. But I couldn't.

So we moved. The house we moved into had suffered a leak from the central heating oil tank, which had soaked into the chalk floor underneath the kitchen. The Army dug progressively deeper holes to try to get rid of the appalling smell, which gave me permanent sinusitis. The disruption to the house meant entertaining was impossible, and we moved at the end of July, when all the toddler activities I was used to going to shut down for the summer. I found it difficult to make new friends, Clive was working very hard, and to top it all I couldn't find a job. I was very miserable and very grouchy. It was July 1990: a few weeks later Saddam Hussein invaded Kuwait.

Clive's workload increased, and he was really needed. He should have been totally fulfilled and happy. He wasn't. His work was classified, and he would not talk about it, but it was obvious that he felt frustrated and at odds with his boss. In February 1991 things came to a head.

Clive had to go for a routine Army medical – the first since he had had the pacemaker fitted. Once again I tried and failed to persuade him to report the pacemaker in advance of the medical. He thought it would be a great joke to turn up for the medical and let the doctor discover the pacemaker. The doctor did not agree. Clive's boss didn't get the joke either. Clive was sent on immediate gardening leave.

The story that came to me via Clive was that the boss had been unhappy with Clive's work for some time, and had decided that the pacemaker and heart problem were the root cause of all Clive's difficulties. Clive had apparently been producing very poor, inappropriate and poorly spelled written work for some time, and had already received several verbal warnings and one written warning. No-one asked why a heart problem should cause problems with writing. Clive was also reported as being stubborn and difficult to manage. Despite this, at a further medical Clive was downgraded one grade medically because of the pacemaker, but no-one looked any further for a medical reason for his difficulties at work. And, of course, he now had a large black mark on his record. Anyone wondering at his stubborn, uncooperative, uncommunicative attitude in the next 18 months looked no further.

We had gone, as a family, to a curry lunch in the mess. The place was quite full, and seating was at a premium. We filled our plates, and looked for somewhere to sit. There was a very large space free, but the Colonel had not yet got food, and that space was very obviously being left clear for him and his wife. My heart sank as Clive headed for it. I tried to point this out, but Clive was having none of it. 'I've as much right to sit there as he has' he declared loudly, and sat down. He was carrying the children's food, so I had little choice but to join him. A few minutes later the Colonel came up, noticed us, and was not best pleased. 'You're sitting in my place', he hissed venomously. Clive refused to budge. Other, more sensible people hastily made space. It did not help our relationship with the people around us.

Clive was sent for another medical, and managed to persuade the doctors that he was very fit, and was graded A2, or whatever such number the Army uses. I don't know if anyone investigated the alleged link between his poor performance at work and the drugs he had been taking for his heart. Anyway, there was no suggestion brought home to me that it was anything other than a personality clash between the Colonel and Clive.

Once his medical status was sorted out, the Army quickly found Clive another job a few miles down the road. He miserably described it as a 'blanket-stacking job'. He was only there for a couple of months, and we were on the move again, back to Oxfordshire and another Army house. This was a more responsible job, with people Clive had worked with before, and he seemed much happier. I was quite surprised when he came home wanting to discuss taking redundancy. The Army was downsizing, and there were some very attractive packages on offer. I didn't like to seem too much like a wet blanket, but I found it very worrying. Clive may not have been particularly happy at work, but it was a steady job with a reasonable income, and we now had two toddlers. I tentatively asked about other jobs. Clive had it all sorted. He would get a job as a teacher – he had a biochemistry degree, and should be able to teach chemistry. We started taking the *Times Literary Supplement*, and checking the pages for likely looking jobs. We talked about moving back to Yorkshire, where we both originally came from, and where we both still had family. Clive put his papers in, and was accepted. He was finally due to leave the Army in September 1992. Whenever I raised the subject of money, he laughed at me. Of course he would get a job; it was just a case of waiting for the right offer to come along. I didn't like to point out that there hadn't been any offers so far.

I don't remember him actually applying for any teaching jobs. The subscription to *Times Literary Supplement*, was cancelled by him. When I queried this, he said he couldn't teach without a teaching certificate, and he was too old to go back to college. Once again, I was surprised. It was not like Clive to decline such a challenge, and he was only 45 – still plenty of time for another career. But he wouldn't be persuaded, and talked of becoming a TEFL (teaching English as a foreign language) teacher, then a security consultant. He even arranged a TEFL course, but managed to arrange it at a time when I had already booked and paid for a diving holiday. It shows how deep the rift between us had grown that I didn't even consider trying to rearrange my diving holiday. I don't think he ever rearranged his course – he certainly never went on it. In the meantime, I had found a job, working part-time for a computer consultancy in Oxford.

Clive was short-listed for a high-profile job with a security firm, for which he had to prepare a talk. The talk was a joint effort – Clive decided what he wanted to say, and I generated overheads on the computer for him to use. He didn't get the job. He was very puzzled because one of the interviewers had asked if he was dyslexic. That was the first real suggestion from someone outside that Clive was having problems with words – why didn't we follow it up?

After that refusal, Clive came home with another suggestion – I should work full-time, and he should be a house-husband. It wasn't exactly what I had had in mind when we started a family, but I could see his point, and it was surely better to have at least one salary coming in. I increased my hours of work, but Clive seemed unable to cope with the house-husband bit.

For step one, Clive decided he had to improve his cooking, and asked me to teach him a few meals that we all enjoyed. I thought the simplest was pasta, bacon and cheese, and carefully explained the recipe to him. He had difficulty understanding some of the instructions, and his idea of bacon pieces 'one inch long' was wide of the mark, but still... He seemed to be getting on OK, so I left him to it, only to be brought back to the kitchen a little later by the smell of burning plastic. Clive had picked up a spatula meant for scraping out cake mix, rather than a fish slice, and was chasing pieces of bacon round the pan with an implement which was steadily melting away in his hands, and coating the pan and the bacon with burnt plastic. Clive hadn't noticed, and seemed very hurt when I insisted on throwing the whole lot out and starting again. His other attempts weren't very much better, and so we compromised on ready meals when it was Clive's turn to cook – more expensive, but at least we ate.

Step two was taking over more child care, but one day I came home from work to find a policeman on the doorstep, holding our three-year-old son Alan by the hand. Clive had taken both children to the swings, and Alan had wandered off – he could move like greased lightning when he wanted to. I never got the complete story, but Alan had been found wandering around his playschool, the other side of a reasonably busy road. I was very concerned, but Clive laughed it off. Whatever might have happened was irrelevant; nothing had happened, and he would be more careful in future. I continued to worry, but really didn't want to give up my job – I was enjoying the work after two years of unemployment, and it was beginning to look as if my salary would soon be the only money coming into the house.

Step three was Clive taking over the washing, but he never got the idea of washing different clothes at different settings – everything went into a hot wash. I soon learned not to put my work clothes into the laundry basket – I had to wash them quietly by hand when Clive was out – and everything else turned a gentle shade of pink. We had just bought a tumble-dryer, as I got sick of wet washing around the house all the time, but it couldn't be installed properly, as we were in a rented house, so every time it was used the vent had to be put through the window. Clive could never remember to do this, so whenever he used the tumble-dryer the whole house filled with steam.

When he cleaned, he was not happy with hoovering round the furniture and dusting the visible surfaces. The Army and his natural habits made him very conscientious and fastidious. Every clean was a spring clean. All the furniture got moved, and all the knick-knacks washed if at all possible. To begin with, most things ended up back in the right places, but as his memory got worse that became less likely. Eventually we would end up with all the furniture at one side of the room, as Clive shifted it all to one side, hoovered that end of the room, moved the furniture to the other side, hoovered the second side, and then put the hoover away and stopped. It was frustrating to come home and have to move things before we could have tea, but at least the house was clean.

I gradually took back most of the jobs, but I kept my office hours up. After all, we would soon be down to the salary from one part-time job.

September came and went with no sign of a job for Clive, and we moved out of the Army house and back into our own – fortunately within reach of Oxford. I increased my hours of work. Clive talked again about becoming a house-husband – the major trouble with that was that he could never remember anything I asked him to do. He was a great cyclist, and went everywhere by bike, but persisted in buying eggs and bringing them home in a rucksack – they rarely survived, but I washed the rucksack, and Clive didn't seem to notice. For Rachel's fifth birthday, she chose a birthday cake from the local shop. I had long since discovered that icing cakes was not one of my strong points – however simple it looked in the book, it proved too complicated for me. The chosen cake was a sponge built up to look like an elegant lady in a crinoline, and Clive offered to collect it on the big day. I was busy trying to organise the party we had arranged, and agreed without really thinking about it. It also came home in a rucksack on a bicycle, with predictable results. I tried to patch it together, but it didn't look quite as good as it had looked in the shop. Fortunately the rest of the party went well, and so we avoided too many tears.

Clive kept on applying for jobs, but I had to help him fill in the application forms. Occasionally he got an interview, but never an offer of a job.

Clive gave a talk to the Rotary Club my brother belonged to. My brother told me the talk had gone very well, but it was a pity there were so many spelling mistakes in the overheads. I couldn't understand that. Clive had given me a travel scrabble set for a wedding present, and we had played many games over the years. He consistently and annoyingly beat me almost all the time – how could he be making elementary spelling mistakes? We watched a French film with subtitles on the TV, and Clive really annoyed me by continually asking for a translation. Again, I couldn't understand it. His French was much better than mine, and there were subtitles in any case. He said he couldn't read the subtitles as he didn't have his contact lenses in, and I believed him. Whenever I read a bed-time story to the children, Clive left the room, and always managed to find an excuse not to read to them himself. I found this inexplicable and very upsetting – it did not occur to me for a long time that he was probably unable to read easily by then.

It wasn't just words and spelling that were difficult. Once we had recognised that Clive's spelling was very erratic, he started bringing all his letters to me for checking. Clive had always done the household admin – he didn't trust my last-minute approach. One day he brought me a cheque he had written to pay a bill. The bill was for one hundred and two pounds; Clive had written a cheque for one thousand and two. He was perplexed at my insistence that he start again. It was a perfectly good cheque, and if it was for more than we owed on this occasion, well, we would just be in credit for a few months. He didn't seem to take on board that the cheque would probably bounce, and, if it did clear, we would have no more money in the account. The idea that the money might run out seemed inconceivable – this from a Yorkshireman who had always known the value of money. I thought once again he was getting at my worry-wort habit, and resolved to worry less in future, but keep a much closer eye on our finances.

When we moved back to our house, we had to buy a few small things, and I decided I wanted some cane waste-paper baskets. I had seen some in a shop in Abingdon, and so when Clive was going shopping I asked him to pick two of these up. I described them quite carefully, told him which shop they were in, and even where in the shop they could be found. Clive nodded agreement, and then came home with a couple of plastic buckets from Woolworths. I probably did weep with frustration and irritation, but Clive was unrepentant. I wanted waste-paper baskets; he had provided receptacles for waste paper, which had the advantage of also being waterproof. I thought he was trying to stop me being so picky and house-proud, and we used the buckets for many years. They didn't quite have the look I had had in mind (when I cared about such things), but they were indeed effective. In later years I got heartily sick of these waste-paper bins, as every doctor Clive saw seemed to think they were very interesting, and showed the difficulties Clive was having with language. That is certainly possible, as his language skills were deteriorating, but I also think it might be that he had disliked being asked to run errands.

The papers before Christmas were full of tokens to collect to get a cheap cross-channel ferry crossing, so you could have a day trip to France and stock up on cheap wine and beer. Clive was very taken with this idea, but he didn't collect any tokens or discuss the idea with me. He just went to the local travel agent and bought a full-price ticket. He then drove to France and bought lots of cheap wine and beer which I had to find storage space for. It all seemed very strange to me, especially since Clive brewed his own beer, and he preferred English bitter to continental lagers. At least the car got him to Calais and home – round about this time every car we owned gave trouble. They were no newer or older than cars we had owned at other times, yet every car stopped working inconveniently and expensively. I can only assume that Clive's very smooth driving style had become rougher and more wearing on engine and gearbox. It was also about this time that I took over the family driving. It was never discussed, and I can't really remember how it happened.

Clive still doggedly continued to look for work, and signed on at the local job centre. I have no idea how he got on with them. He should have been entitled to a little unemployment benefit, but he persisted in taking a job an old colleague offered him, which offered a few hours' work in London two or three times a month. The pay never paid the expenses he incurred travelling to and from London, and of course each time he worked he signed off benefit. So whatever he may have been entitled to we never got. The redundancy payment diminished with alarming speed, but Clive shouted at me whenever I mentioned it. He would get a job, he was certain. He rang me at work one day to tell me that he had been offered a job – when I got home I looked at the letter and he had actually been sent an application form. But Clive always put up a good front – he always had a reasonable explanation, and I was too busy to take much notice by now. Conversations with Clive seemed quite pointless. Whatever we decided, he'd ignore it and do whatever he wanted, so I just let him get on with things, and tried to keep the rest of the family going. Every Friday he bought a local paper, and we would spread it on the floor and go through the jobs section looking for possibilities. I'd help him fill out the application form, and he got a few interviews, but never anything more.

Finally, he was offered a job, as a security consultant with a firm in Yorkshire. The job was very close to his mother's house, so he arranged to go up and stay with her, and see how things got on. If it worked out, we would look for a house up there. He lasted three days, and was sent home in a hurry. The firm never told him why they didn't find his work satisfactory; they found it 'too embarrassing'. They also never paid him. Unfortunately, while he was there, his bicycle was stolen.

After his redundancy from the Army, Clive joined the Territorial Army (TA) and went on weekend training exercises with them, probably about once a month. I never heard how he got on until there was a two-week exercise down at the coast. Clive was sent home early, and a letter to me (this was the first time the Army had contacted me) explained that this was because he was becoming a 'laughing stock'. I didn't consider the letter closely, and can't reproduce it now – it ended up in shreds in the rubbish. I tore it into pieces the size of a postage stamp, and, when I couldn't tear the pieces any smaller, I took scissors to them. A few days later I got a telephone call asking me (not Clive) what was going on, and a few days after that a letter from the TA dispensing with Clive's services after 23 years in the Army. No advice about any possible change in his pension entitlement was offered.

Just after this he admitted to me that he was having problems with reading and writing, and asked me to start accompanying him on the hospital visits. His story was very confusing – like everything at this time. He had apparently already been to see one specialist, who couldn't find anything wrong and referred him on to a neurologist. It was all very complicated, and I can't go back to get the full story from Clive's hospital notes, as they were lost without trace.

Clive and I went to a consultation with the neurologist. The story of Clive and the waste-paper baskets was discussed at length, as were the egg-shopping trips. Clive was referred for a series of neuropsychological tests – as far as I could see, mostly pen and paper tests taking about an hour each. I would meet Clive, deliver him to the hospital (he was not by now reliable about getting to a definite place at a definite time, and the hospital was very close to where I was working), sometimes wait for him and sometimes go for a walk, then collect him and see him safely on his way home. On one occasion there was a fire alarm, and so the three of us sat outside in the summer sunshine, and naturally talked about what the tests showed. At least, the subject seemed a natural one to me. The person doing the testing – a very nice young psychologist – got very upset, and said that she should not have to give us the results of the tests – that was up to the neurologist. But it was clear that Clive was doing very badly in some of the tests, and that his problems were not confined to any particular area. Because of his pacemaker, Clive couldn't have an MRI scan, but he did have a CT scan (a type of X-ray), which didn't show anything amiss. He also had a lumbar puncture, where a needle is used to extract some of the fluid surrounding the brain and spinal column. Lumbar punctures are notorious for generating headaches, and the standard instruction is to take life very easy for a few days after the test to give the body time to replace the fluid. Clive interpreted this in his own inimitable way: he had cycled to the hospital for the test (I don't know where I was on this particular day), so after it he cycled home – six miles, up and down a very steep hill – and then he hoovered the house. I came home to find him sitting down complaining of a slight headache. The next day he got up as usual at 5:30 a.m., cycled to the pool and went for a swim. Then he cycled home. I told him what an idiot I thought he was, and tried to persuade him to go to bed and lie flat. He refused, but eventually allowed me to ring the GP. She was sufficiently concerned to come out and see him, and ordered him to his bed to *lie flat*. He was prepared to follow her instructions, and downstairs she signed a sick note for him – the first of many. It was the first time he admitted he was unfit for work. I remember the date – it was 15 October 1993 – Clive's 46th birthday.

With hindsight

How could I have been so blind? Clive's behaviour was so different from earlier, and things he had always managed competently were now beyond him. The truth is that things changed so slowly and gradually that each step seemed perfectly reasonable. People do have conflicts with their boss. Husbands can forget they have promised to babysit on a particular night; they have been known to forget their wife's birthday. Dementia is very rare in those under 65; most GPs won't see one case in their career. And Clive, after the very early stages, never admitted he was having difficulties; indeed, he became very good at hiding any problems. But our life could have been so much better if his illness had been recognised earlier. All the fights and arguments could have been avoided. We could have had three more good years together, and made the most of Clive's time with his children. If Clive's illness had been diagnosed in 1989, before the problems with the Army, we could have made the most of the time we had left together, instead of spending a lot of it in irritation, misunderstanding and misery. And our finances would have been much healthier.

I attended a conference not very long ago when one of the speakers, an American geriatrician, said he was against giving people a very early diagnosis. He explained that to give a diagnosis of 'possible early dementia' would stigmatise the people concerned, affecting their relationship with everyone around them, might stop them driving and would generally make their lives much more difficult, without in any way helping them. I wanted to ask him about an early diagnosis for younger people, people with a job, a mortgage and possibly a young dependent family. An early diagnosis for them might mean retirement on grounds of ill health and a pension, rather than the sack and a life of poverty. But I never got the chance – the conference was very busy, and I could never catch his eye. Sure, dementia is very difficult to diagnose even when it is quite far advanced, but there are conditions with similar symptoms which are treatable, and even, if the eventual diagnosis is dementia, it makes subsequent life much more comfortable if the person with dementia is able to take medical retirement, and keep the pension they are entitled to. It also gives them time to make other arrangements and, if they wish, make such things as a living will.

Even with hindsight, I find it difficult to see what I could have done differently. Things changed so slowly, and the initial symptoms were so nebulous. It never occurred to me to try and see my husband's GP. I didn't realise that there was a medical problem. In fact, I still have difficulty understanding an illness that can cause someone to forget how to spell. At the time, Clive was registered with an Army doctor, so my seeing him would have had implications for Clive's work, and in any case I would not have expected him to see me. Perhaps I could have gone to my own GP, but I already seemed to spend far too much time there with the minor accidents and illnesses of two toddlers. I didn't have any close friends I felt able to confide in, and I felt very much like a nagging wife. In fact, for a long time I wondered if the problem was mine and not Clive's. I didn't even talk to Clive's or my family. It was impossible to raise such a topic over the phone. When I finally allowed myself to confide in a close friend, I felt as if I had betrayed Clive in even admitting to such doubts.

I was frustrated and very worried for most of this time. Clive used to say that if I didn't have something to worry about I would worry about the things I didn't know that I ought to worry about. Again, hindsight is wonderfully clear, but what was most disturbing about this time was that Clive wasn't at all worried about the things that were wrong. That insouciance, that calm acceptance of things, that inability to see the consequences of one's actions, is very much a symptom of his illness.

What is clear to me now is that if I had recognised that the difficulties I was having communicating with Clive were not just mine, and that the people he worked with were having similar difficulties, the last ten years of Clive's life could have been much easier and happier.

Chapter 2

The Old Clive

It's a beautiful spring day in early May 1970, the first Saturday in term. A few days ago Clive and I were walking in the fields around my parents' Yorkshire home, and for the only time in my life I saw hares boxing. Today Clive is going to take me punting. I rest back on the cushions as he steers the punt out from the backwater where it is moored, and onto the river Cherwell. The sun is warm on my back, but, when I trail a hand in the water, the river is still very cold. Clive looks very handsome, water dripping off his arms as he grips the pole – 12 feet of polished wood with a metal fork at one end. The backwater is very shallow, and the pole only goes down a foot or two, but when we get to the Cherwell the water is much deeper, and Clive has to squat to keep hold of the end. He makes the punting look so easy: as he rises from the squat he throws the pole in the air, and catches it near the middle, ready for the next stroke. 'Splosh' goes the pole in the water, and Clive's hands climb up the wood as he pushes the punt along. Then he pulls the pole off the bottom and trails it in the water for a few seconds before starting the whole process again. The Cherwell is lined with willow trees which are just coming into leaf; the daffodils in the Parks are beginning to die, and a few families of ducklings are out on the river for their first view of the wide world. We go under the Rainbow Bridge, its high arch especially designed to allow punts to pass underneath. It is too early in the season for there to be many other boats about, and we have the river almost to ourselves. The sun is so warm, and Clive's punting so hypnotic, I almost fall asleep, but decide to be energetic instead, and have a go at punting. We change places with the punt wobbling rather alarmingly, and now Clive is sitting down facing me, and I am standing at the end with the pole in my hands. It is very heavy, and I settle for a much less elegant movement as I shuffle my hands up the pole ready to drop it vertically into the river. While Clive seems to have stayed dry apart from his forearms, I am soon soaked as muddy river water drains down my arms and body. When Clive punts, the pole stays close to the side of the punt, and there is one long smooth forward movement. Alas, as I push the pole it parts company with the side of the punt. We are not moving up the river, but heading diagonally across towards the bank. Clive gets the paddle ready to fend off a hawthorn bush, and push us back to the centre of the river, while giving me instructions to steer using the pole as a rudder. I do my inelegant shuffle down the pole, and try again. This time I manage a few strokes before we head bankwards again, and get entangled in the branches of a willow tree. We're both almost helpless with laughter as we seem well caught – Clive can push us off with the paddle, but it is very difficult to disentangle the pole. A bit later, and I am feeling much more in control. A long stroke pushes the punt forward, and I give the pole a good tug, getting ready for the next stroke. I am beginning to think I might even try Clive's elegant throw, and am not paying attention to things. The pole remains stuck in the river. I keep hold, but the punt is moving on, and the pole with me attached is not. 'Let go now' says Clive. He doesn't shout, but the authority in his voice is unmistakeable. I let go of the pole. The punt floats gently on with the pole stuck in the mud behind us. Thanks to Clive, I have avoided the 'monkey on a stick' trick beloved of spectators, which invariably ends with the monkey in the river. We retrieve the pole, and Clive punts us home. It has been a magical afternoon.

I met Clive at the end of my first term at Oxford University. I had gone along with a friend to the University Judo Club, and Clive was the instructor; his judo jacket had pulled loose, he was bathed in sweat, and had sweat dripping off his nose. We joined in, and the class was so intensive that, despite the stretches at the end, the next day I could hardly move. I was not initially impressed. But I had the Christmas vacation to recover, and next term I joined the judo club. It was a friendly class, and necessarily quite small because of the space available, so Clive and I soon got talking. We discovered that we both came from Yorkshire, and our families lived only a few miles apart. In the Easter vacation we made arrangements to go walking in the Dales. Clive could drive, and had access to a car, both of which made a great impression on me. He picked me up one morning, and in the excitement I left without my walking boots; something I realised after a few miles. I had to confess, and ask Clive to go back. Such a confession in my family would have been met by heavy sighs, muttered comments about even Oxford undergraduates being pretty stupid, and the return home would have taken place in an icy silence. Clive hooted with laughter, turned the car round, and continued to talk about where we could go for the day. I found it a refreshing change, and I think that was when I started to fall in love.

I was in my first year of a physics degree; Clive was in the last year of biochemistry. Clive was not a natural academic; he was a very active member of the Army Officer Training Corps and a mainstay of the judo club. Most days he would drop round for a cup of tea after a day spent revising. The biochemistry library had an excellent view of the RAF parachute training school at

Weston-on-the-Green, and Clive could always tell me how the jumping was going. He didn't tell me how the revising was going, but it was clear to me that Clive was forcing himself to study a subject he really had no interest in. He had access to a college punt, and we spent many afternoons and evenings out on the river – his friends described Clive in a punt as a 'motorised speed-boat'. Clive and I had a fairly competitive relationship. One weekend I got roped in to organising a judo match. We had to move all the mats from the small judo room to a bigger room up a flight of stairs. The mats were heavy and the rooms some way apart, but neither of us was prepared to be the first to ask for a break, so we moved the mats in record time.

Clive's exams were before mine, so he had a few days free. He was always energetic and keen to keep fit; one of the crazy ideas he had at this time was to walk for 24 hours and see how far he could go. He set out early one summer morning, and about an hour later turned up as I was having breakfast in college. He explained that his boots were rubbing, and so he could see the exercise was pointless. I would have felt obliged to continue until I had at least a couple of blisters to show, but that was not Clive's way. He never felt the need to explain his actions.

After college he applied to join the Army. We met in York the day he had his Army entrance medical. We walked round the walls in glorious sunshine, and then went to the cinema. I got my times mixed up and missed the last train home, so Clive borrowed his mother's car and took me home. It was a different world then. I couldn't telephone my parents and explain that I would be late, as we had no telephone.

Clive was accepted for the Army, and joined the Parachute Regiment. He came to see me just before he joined up, and we agreed that there was nothing serious between us; he was serious about his Army career, and I about my degree, so we staged a 'parting is such sweet sorrow' scene, and he went off to Aldershot. Actually I was fibbing – I very much enjoyed Clive's company, and was not looking forward to not seeing him any more. But I did have a lot to look forward to, including going back to Oxford, so my pride kept me from telling Clive any of this. If he didn't want to be with me, then so be it.

A few weeks later I went back to Oxford, only to discover that Clive was stationed at Abingdon, a few miles south of Oxford, for several weeks of parachute training. October in England is not the best of parachuting weather, so Clive had quite a lot of free time, and spent much of it in Oxford with me. 'Hah' I thought. So much for not wanting to see me any more. In January Clive went off to do the Parachute Regiment's 'P Company'. The Paras have always prided themselves on their level of fitness, and 'P Company' was the start of this. For several weeks Clive was running up hills and making long marches in the Brecon Beacons, always carrying a very heavy rucksack. He came back for a couple of weekends and sent me off to raid Marks and Spencers for large-size tights and long johns; it was a very cold winter, and I think he had a fairly miserable time. Certainly he was never prepared to come walking in the Brecons with me afterwards.

Sometime during that time, when Clive was doing his training, and visiting me whenever he was free, the relationship became serious, at least as far as I was concerned. While Clive was at Oxford he was rather like a fish that was trying to learn how to fly. Once he joined the Army, he was in his natural element, much more relaxed and self-confident, and I got to know him better. He was always a very quiet person, but we shared a weird sense of humour, and he was honest, straightforward and reliable. We both came from Yorkshire, and we felt united against the Southerners.

Clive was different from all the other students I knew. I was a physics student – one of 20 or so women in a group of 200 – and my main hobbies then were judo and climbing, both male-dominated, so I knew plenty of other men. I was a bit of a tomboy, but Clive seemed to like and approve of this, whereas many of the others didn't. I liked his friends and he got on well with mine; we were just very compatible. And he was very sexy. I never really thought about his looks, but one day we were out together and met a friend of mine who hadn't seen Clive before. She commented on how handsome he was, and when I looked again I was forced to agree.

P Company confirmed Clive in his determination to keep himself very fit. Every day after that, wherever we were posted, and whatever the weather, he ran for at least an hour every day. He also cycled to work if at all possible (and he was prepared to cycle further, and on busier roads than many). Once he had completed P Company, he joined the second battalion of the Parachute Regiment as a second lieutenant, and was soon off to Belfast – it being 1971 and pretty much the height of the Troubles. I visited him once, in the middle of his four-month tour, and was privileged to see the vulnerable side of his character. He clung to me as I imagine a drowning man would grab a raft. It shows the stress he was under at the time, as I was never allowed a similar glimpse afterwards, even when he was ill. Clive prided himself on being cool, rational and self-sufficient. He wasn't the cold fish that sounds, though. He just reckoned he had failed if he showed anger or fear. I came back from that trip wearing an engagement ring.

He visited me at the end of his four-month tour in Ireland. It was November, and children were still allowed to buy bangers and set them off in the street. A couple of days after he got back, we were out walking when there was a bang. I looked around, and then realised that Clive was no longer next to me – he had taken immediate evasive action, and jumped behind a wall. At the time I thought it was funny. It was only later that I realised how different Clive's life in the Army was from my sheltered existence as an Oxford undergraduate.

Clive had four tours in Northern Ireland in the next two years. In between tours, he was based in Aldershot. One tour was followed by a 'jolly' of two weeks in Jamaica. He was part of a team doing a presentation free-fall parachute display into the football stadium. Unfortunately the wind was rather stronger than expected, and some of the team missed the stadium. Clive would never tell me if he was one of these. I met him at Brize Norton when he came home, with a broken front tooth. He had dived into a very clear stream which wasn't quite as deep as he had hoped, and crunched his mouth. Clive never did things by halves. He hadn't just chipped the tooth; he'd actually broken it just beyond the gum-line, and the nerve was showing. This was just before the return flight, so he had taken a couple of aspirin and got on the plane. The pain from his tooth must have been agonising, but I am sure it never occurred to Clive to make a fuss and possibly delay his flight back.

We became engaged in the summer of my second year, and married a year later. I hadn't forgotten my hopes for a career. I just assumed that I could have both. I was by this time very much in love, and wanted to be with Clive whatever else happened. Nowadays we would probably have lived together, but that wasn't an option then, especially for an Army officer. Things nearly came unstuck before they started. We had planned to get married in the middle of August, but the Army sent Clive off to Ireland at very short notice. He thought that was a hilarious joke; I was less amused, and we had a blazing row by telephone and letter. But we made it up before he came home, and finally got married a month later. We always argued about the date. I thought it was the 16th, and Clive thought it was the 17th. We finally thought of looking at the silver cigarette box that was the traditional present from Clive's colleagues, although neither of us smoked, and Clive was right as usual. I don't know why I ever bothered arguing. Clive was almost always right.

I stayed in Oxford and embarked on a research degree, and Clive lived in Aldershot and visited most weekends. We took up free-fall parachuting, and spent the weekends at Weston-on-the-Green, waiting for the clouds to clear or the wind to drop. When everything came together, free-fall was a great feeling. We went skiing at Christmas, and life was good.

After four years in the Parachute Regiment, Clive applied to transfer to the Royal Army Ordnance Corps, with the intention of training as an ammunition specialist and bomb-disposal officer. He had worked with the bomb squad in Northern Ireland, and been inspired. It was by no means certain that he would be accepted. There had been a high casualty rate in the early days of the Troubles, and the Army had brought in very strict selection tests, including a psychological questionnaire. Clive couldn't quite see what his appreciation of pushing his feet into furry slippers had to do with his ability to handle ammunition, but he obviously supplied the right answers, as he was accepted for training. He went off to Warwickshire; I had decided by now that physics research was not for me, and had found a job near Aldershot, but was soon sent off to a project in Scotland. Fortunately Clive had some leave before his course, and we spent a happy month climbing Scottish mountains and fighting midges off.

After the ammunition training, Clive was posted to Germany – a long way from the Scottish Highlands in the days before cheap flights, so I joined him out there. I managed to find work with a German company, learned German, and developed a taste for exploring different places and cultures. The Army then sent Clive off again, this time back to Northern Ireland as a bomb-disposal officer. He never talked about his time there, making it very clear it was all covered by the Official Secrets Act. Even now his colleagues are very reticent in public, but I came across some photos of his bomb-disposal activities much later, when I was clearing things out, and I was very glad Clive had not had an accident. Clive regarded it as one of the high points of his life: he was doing the job he had trained for, his work was appreciated and worthwhile, and he was part of a very select group.

We had kept up free-fall as a hobby even after Clive left the Paras, but Clive was posted back to the UK, and free-fall in the UK was both very expensive and very frustrating – many weekends were washed out because of low cloud, too much wind, or no aeroplane. We were looking for an alternative sport, and the diving club was looking for recruits, so we joined up. Our first dive was in a cold, muddy English gravel pit, but then we went on holiday to Gibraltar and I was hooked. Clive was never as keen as I was, but he came along to keep me company. We went down to Portsmouth to order wet-suits; it was Saturday and we had been measured for suits by mid-morning. Clive suddenly announced he had always fancied seeing if he could run a marathon; there was one on the Isle of Wight that afternoon, and did I mind if he took the ferry across and ran in it? It was the first I had heard of this ambition but certainly not the last. He ran one every few weeks for the next two years, and his fastest time was three hours and one minute. He was always hoping to shave off that last minute in his next marathon, but he never managed it.

It seems worth noting that in all this time Clive was hardly ever ill, not even a cold. I had appendicitis, bronchitis, a dislocated thumb from a skiing holiday, and a whole host of minor injuries and illnesses, but I can only remember Clive being ill once, with the flu. Not bad for 15 years.

Clive was selected for the Army Staff Course – a year-long training course at Camberley for potential high flyers. By now he had been promoted to Major, and seemed to have a glittering career ahead of him. After Camberley, Clive was given a staff job in London. He hated the commuting, and he hated the job. He was working on plans to reinforce the Army on the Rhine in the event of a Russian invasion (this was still during the Cold War). He thought it was a waste of time, and was convinced that we ought to be much more worried about the threat from terrorist groups. Still, his friends in the postings branch hadn't forgotten him; after a few months of this we were on the move again. The United Arab Emirates (UAE) Army had requested the loan of an ammunition specialist, and off to Dubai we went.

We arrived in the middle of summer, and temperatures hit 48 degrees Celsius on our first day. Clive was off to work the next day. He was very keen to hit the ground running, and he had a lot to get to grips with. He had responsibility for 150 men and the purchase, storage, use and subsequent disposal of all the ammunition for the Dubai arm of the UAE Defence Force. Although many people spoke English, the working language was Arabic, which Clive managed to pick up very quickly.

I was left to my own devices, but soon made contact with the local diving club, and started to teach diving. Every Friday I was out diving, and Clive often joined me. When my diving students qualified to dive in the sea, we took them out to a wreck that had been sunk to attract fish. I followed the book, and took my students cautiously around the outside of the wreck. I learned some time later that Clive was not so timid. He took his buddies through the wreck, and through a door that clanged ominously behind them. There was in fact another way out, and the entire route was safe, but whenever I went through there the 'bong' reverberated alarmingly. None of Clive's buddies ever complained, and there was competition to dive with him rather than me.

We were in Dubai during the forgotten Gulf War between the Iraqis and the Iranians. It didn't affect us much in Dubai, although, as Clive rarely talked about his work, I don't know how his job was affected. Clive came home in some discomfort one day, and eventually told me he had spent the day out in the Gulf. An oil tanker had been hit by a missile which had not exploded, and Clive had been disposing of the missile by cutting a hole in the side of the tanker and gently tipping the missile into the sea. The discomfort came from the size of boiler suit he had been lent to protect his own clothes; they only had extra-small. It was the first and last I heard of the more active side of his job; if he talked at all about his job it was about the office work and the people he was working with.

We both loved Dubai. When Clive's tour there finished, he was asked to stay on and transfer to the Dubai services. It was a very difficult decision, but neither of us wanted to settle there for a long time; we liked the freedom and mobility that came with Clive's job in the British Army. We also both expected that his career would continue to progress, and were beginning to think about starting a family. When we came back to the UK I confidently expected things to keep on getting better, as they had done so far.

With hindsight

I didn't expect things to last forever, but I did hope for longer than we had...

Chapter 3

Diagnosis

We're standing by the roadside outside a wildlife park in Kenya. The sun is beating down; it is the middle of summer here. We have just spent the week on board a boat, diving around the islands off the Kenyan coast. This is the wash-out day; you need to allow 24 hours between diving and flying in order to avoid decompression sickness. The people at the hotel had suggested the park which has been created out of an old open-cast mining area. Huge ammonites three feet across litter the paths. When we sat down in the café for an orange juice, a gibbon whizzed out of the trees, knocked mine over, and lapped up the spillage, with me fascinated a few inches away. The hotel staff had been very keen to book us a taxi and driver for the day, and it wouldn't have been very expensive, but, when he heard it was possible to go on the bus, Clive had decided immediately that that was what we would do. We had been dropped off in town, wandered round the market, and then caught a bus with no difficulty — the bus started from there, so we just turned up at the right place and waited. I was beginning to get worried that getting back would not be so easy. We had been here for nearly an hour, and several buses had zoomed past, ignoring our gentle waves. I looked at Clive, but there was no help there. He wore his very familiar, slightly bemused expression. Finally a local took pity on us. When the next bus came, he waved vigorously, then jumped up and down. The bus stopped, and we managed to squeeze on. The local vanished – I never even managed to give him a tip. The bus delivered us to the market place, where I found a taxi to take us back to the hotel. There was a lesson here – I could no longer rely on Clive to sort things out for me.

Clive had been seeing a neurologist in Oxford, and had been referred on for several sessions of neuropsychological tests. Some time in November the neurologist rang me to arrange a time when we could discuss the results of all the tests. He called me at work, so I arranged a time a few days later.

It was a difficult conversation for both of us, and very short. He had a rotten cold, and it was the end of a long day. I had foolishly asked him to ring me after I had finished work for the day, and so had spent the entire day waiting for the call. I now know that sort of attitude is called denial. I just thought I was trying to keep my private life and my work life separate. I doubt if we were on the phone for longer than two minutes. He told me that my husband had pre-senile dementia, that he would send details to my GP, that he was sorry, goodbye. I sort of expected an appointment to see him for further details, and to be able to ask questions, but it never came. He never told Clive, but left that job to me.

I know I was in the office when the call came, and I know my boss was there as well, but I have blanked out everything else about that evening. I must have said at least a few words to my boss – it must have been obvious I had had some devastating news. I can't remember getting home. I must have done, driving the car on auto-pilot. I must have prepared dinner, then bathed the children, read a bed-time story and got them to bed, then cooked another dinner for Clive and me. I must have done, because I always did, and certainly no-one else would have done, but I can't remember any of it. I probably went back into the office the next day, and sat at a desk and stared at a computer screen, but it is all blanked out in my mind. It was November 1993. Clive had been out of work for over a year. Our children were four and five.

'Pre-senile dementia' – it didn't mean much to me. I got the dictionary out. 'Dementia – the usually progressive deterioration of intellectual functions such as memory that can occur while other brain functions such as those controlling movement and the senses are retained. From the Latin *de* away + *ment* mind.' 'Senile – occurring in or believed to be characteristic of later life.' 'Pre – prefix, before, earlier.' What a dreadful diagnosis to give someone second-hand, with no follow-up or hand-holding. There was then no treatment available, and the neurologist evidently felt he had done his best by delivering the diagnosis, but I still think it is no way to treat anyone. And, alas, it subsequently became very clear that a lot of people considered a diagnosis of dementia meant the person with the diagnosis ceased to be a person at all.

In many ways, the diagnosis came as a relief. The faint suspicion that there was something wrong had grown stronger and stronger over the previous weeks, months and years. At last we knew there were real problems, with a real cause and a real name. We had some idea of how things might develop. It wasn't a very cheerful picture, but not as bad as my nightmares. Armed with a diagnosis, we could face the world outside – employers, friends, teachers, family – with a reason for the way things were.

The consultant had referred us back to our GP, so a few days later we were in our GP's surgery. We walked in together. Almost before he sat down, Clive put on his best, jocular, no-nonsense Army officer voice. 'Well', he boomed 'so how long have I got, then?' The GP looked as though someone had hit her with a sledgehammer. Clive had no idea of the impact he had had. I don't know how much was Clive putting up a good front, and how much the illness had robbed him of the sense of what was said. She explained the reasons for the diagnosis, talked about a research project at Oxford that might be able to give us some more information, mentioned the Alzheimer's Society, and we left. It was the first of many visits, and she was always supportive and helpful.

My mother lived in Yorkshire, two hundred miles away, but we were very close. My father had died 18 months before Rachel was born, and my mother had spent a lot of time with us when the children were babies. I cried on the phone to her as I told her the news. She often told me later how shocked she had been, and how she wished I could have told her in person. None of that came across to me at the time. She was already coming to stay with us for Christmas. She offered to stay on for two or three weeks so that Clive and I could have a holiday together.

I cried in front of my boss as I told him the reason I had stayed late in the office the other day. I cried in front of my colleagues when they offered sympathy. I cried in front of the children's headmaster when I told him. I cried on Clive's shoulder. I don't remember Clive ever crying on my shoulder. How much was the natural Clive, how much was the self-control the Army had taught him, how much was family background, and how much was the illness flattening his understanding of what was happening to him, I shall never know. Clive may have been putting up a good front, but I started on a crying jag that lasted for two or three years. It wasn't something I seemed to have any control over, and it was something I am still somewhat ashamed of. So much for my 'stiff upper lip'.

Clive's mother still lived in Yorkshire, and his brother and sister also lived a long way from us. Nonetheless, they were a very close family, with several phone calls exchanged each week. Clive didn't want to tell his family; he 'didn't want to worry them'. I tried to persuade him that they were probably already worried, and that if they hadn't already noticed things were amiss they were bound to quite soon. Clive was adamant. I 'ummed and arred' for a few days, and, after one very awkward phone call, decided that I was incapable of lying to them, and unwilling to try, and that cutting off all contact was a worse alternative. They had to know. So I wrote three very difficult letters to his mother, sister and brother, my tears dripping onto the computer keyboard. Of course they had realised something was wrong, and like me they were at least happy to have a name to give to what was going on. Clive's brother was a doctor, and he advised us to ask for a second opinion. We were referred to a London hospital which specialises in younger people with dementia. They sent us an appointment for January – the Oxford research project agreed to see Clive in December.

In the meantime, the normal family life had to continue. Children had to be fed and got to school, clothes had to be washed, and shopping and housework had to be done. My mind split into several independent compartments. I even managed to put in some productive time in the office. Clive continued to occupy himself, as he had done for the previous year. At least he no longer had to search the local and national papers for a likely looking job, then try and get an application form, fill it in and send it off. He finally allowed himself to admit that this process was beyond him. I wish he had done so sooner. I wish the Army had tried to discover why he was having such difficulty for the last 18 months of his time with them. How much easier life would have been for us all, and how much more we could have enjoyed Clive's last few years with us.

We saw OPTIMA (the Oxford Project to Investigate Memory and Ageing) for the first time on 15 December 1993. OPTIMA is a research project which started in 1988 – the team invited elderly people with and without Alzheimer's disease in for a whole set of physical and cognitive tests, which were repeated every six months for those with Alzheimer's, and yearly for those without. The aim was to see how the illness progressed, and how the 'normal elderly' changed as well. Fortunately for us, in the early 1990s they also decided to recruit some younger people with dementia, and Clive was invited to join them. We spent the whole day there; Clive had lots of tests and scans, and for the first time someone talked to me without Clive. Up till then, we had always been seen together, and I had found this very frustrating. We would walk in, and the doctor would ask how things were. 'Oh, fine, just fine' Clive would say, and there was absolutely no way I could express my fears and frustrations. Especially as Clive had been rejected for job after job, in front of him I felt I had to be supportive.

I was seen by one of the OPTIMA nurses while Clive was seen by the doctors. For the first time, I was given advice about things we should do to help organise the future the way we wanted it – power of attorney, wills, applying for benefits and pensions. I cried a lot that day as well. Although OPTIMA is a research project, they provide a lot of support to their participants, and support was what Clive and I needed right then. It was such a relief to be able to express my worries about the future, and be reassured that we were not alone.

The 'pre-senile dementia' neurologist Clive had seen had taken a CT scan of Clive's brain in May. The CT scan showed some very mild atrophy in Clive's brain tissue. OPTIMA repeated the scan in December, and saw more marked atrophy. Whatever process was destroying Clive's brain tissue was progressing quite fast. OPTIMA also carried out a SPECT scan – this involves measuring the uptake of radioactive water in the brain, and shows the blood supply to the brain. Even to my non-medical eye, it was very clear that there were huge areas of Clive's brain that were using very little oxygen. These were principally in the parts of the brain that control language and memory, but there were also big holes in the frontal lobes. When I looked at the results of the tests, I was not surprised at the difficulties Clive was having – instead I was very impressed at how well he was managing.

OPTIMA's diagnosis was that Clive had semantic dementia, and also 'probable' Alzheimer's disease. Armed with that, we went home and prepared to celebrate Christmas. My mother came down from Yorkshire, and we had a fairly quiet Christmas at

home with just the five of us. Then we went to stay with Clive's
sister for a few days, and met the entire Beaumont clan. It was the
first time we had seen most of our extended family since the
diagnosis. It was quite a good Christmas, all things considered.

In the New Year, Clive and I went away on a diving holiday. I
had put a lot of effort into finding somewhere where the sun
would shine, and the water would be warm, and we had a
wonderful holiday in Kenya. We were on a fairly small diving
boat, and on the first evening the captain asked me what was
wrong with Clive. His question came as quite a shock. For so
long, I had been convinced that there was something wrong with
Clive, and very few other people seemed to agree with me. It had
been a relief to me that his family had noticed how changed he
was. This was the first time a stranger had noticed anything. We
had a great time, though we were not great company for the other
people on the boat. The sun shone, the water was warm, and the
diving was good. I had booked the trip at very short notice, and
so we were travelling business class; on the flight home we were
moved up to first class, and came home in great style. For the first
part of the journey I could see the river Nile below us – a winding
line in the midst of the desert. A telephone cricket had crept into
one of our diving bags, and for a couple of nights after we got
back his distinctive chirping could be heard.

He was still chirping the morning we set out for Clive's
appointment at the National Hospital for Neurology and Neurosurgery in London. Again, Clive was taken off for tests, and I was
asked in great detail about the events that had brought us to see
them. They conducted some different tests – they didn't repeat
any of the scans, as they could use the results from OPTIMA, but
they were testing for the rarer dementias. I'm told that one of the
tests is to discuss common proverbs with people. If you ask a
normal person what the saying 'too many cooks spoil the broth'
means, they will probably talk about how having too many
people trying to do one job will end in failure. People with
frontal-lobe dementia are more likely to be less general, and will

talk about several people putting salt into a pot of soup. And if you give someone with frontal-lobe dementia a pair of spectacles, they are likely to put them on, whereas normal people will hand them back. At the end of the day came a diagnosis of frontal-lobe dementia, probably Pick's disease.

These were pre-internet days, so I spent time in the next few weeks haunting the Oxford libraries, fortunately a fruitful hunting ground. Frontal-lobe dementia, as you might expect, affects the frontal lobes of the brain – the bits immediately behind the forehead. This is the area of the brain that is most developed in humans, and governs 'executive function' – the ability to plan ahead, to see the consequences of one's actions and then to act appropriately. People with Pick's disease have specific abnormalities in this part of the brain, and also defects in the brain areas governing speech and language. But the books mentioned how the speech could be severely disturbed, and yet number skills retained. This did not apply to Clive – he had started having difficulties with numbers at about the same time his spelling mistakes started.

Every book mentioned the 'slow and insidious onset' – that certainly applied to Clive. Speech problems and personality changes were also common, and no book was prepared to give any likely timescale for the illness. All agreed it was progressive and eventually fatal, with probably a complete loss of speech eventually. I did lots more crying, but finally decided to try and forget it all, and just get on with making the most of every day. One thing all the doctors agreed on was that Clive's illness was just bad luck. Although some types of early onset dementia do run in families, there was no suggestion that this might be the case for Clive. Hardly the silver lining that is said to hide behind every cloud, but better news than it could have been, especially for his brother and sister, and all our children.

With hindsight

Diagnosing dementia is very difficult. The first step is to decide that cognitive functions are affected in several areas – things like reading, writing, calculating, short-term memory (remembering what someone told you five minutes ago) – and that this is an ongoing problem. The next step is to rule out all the other causes for similar symptoms, some of which are treatable. Such conditions include depression (which was my GP's initial diagnosis), thyroid problems, vitamin B12 deficiency and hydrocephalus. But cognitive abilities vary hugely from person to person, so an early diagnosis can be very difficult if the impairment is not great. CT and MRI scans can show some changes in the brain structure, but these are often only apparent quite late in the illness. Some types of dementia also give rise to physical symptoms, especially in fine motor control, so a finger-tapping test is often included. And, even when reached, a diagnosis of 'dementia' is only a very broad description of symptoms. There are many illnesses which cause dementia, and distinguishing between them is even more difficult. For Clive, we started out with a diagnosis of 'pre-senile dementia' – the pre-senile merely means that Clive was under 65 when symptoms started. The next diagnosis was 'probable Alzheimer's disease with semantic dementia', indicating difficulties with short-term memory which were getting worse over time, and semantic dementia – problems with understanding and using words. Then from London came a diagnosis of 'frontal-lobe dementia, probably Pick's disease', indicating difficulties with language, and also changes in character and loss of executive function. The final diagnosis from the post-mortem was 'cortico-basal dementia'. All these diagnoses came from highly respected doctors. Clive spent many hours doing test after test, and I think the variation shows how difficult such diagnoses are. The only accurate diagnosis comes from a look at the affected brain tissue, and taking a brain biopsy is not acceptable unless it can lead to an effective treatment.

Fortunately there are no futile 'I wish…' points here for me. Once we had the initial diagnosis, we were very lucky. The OPTIMA project accepted Clive as a patient, and they gave us invaluable advice about how to cope as the illness progressed – more on this later in the book. Our GP agreed to our request for a second opinion, and we were seen quickly by a consultant who is world-renowned in the field of younger onset dementia. The hospital in London was about to start a support group for relatives of those with Pick's disease, which again gave me a lot of advice and support. We also received excellent support and advice from our GP.

However, I get very angry when I think about the way the initial diagnosis was given to us. I understand that the neurologist was very busy, and that he did not feel he had any more to offer us beyond the diagnosis, but he should at least have seen Clive to tell him. Clive was quite capable of understanding the diagnosis, though fortunately I think he could no longer imagine the implications, and I think the consultant was in a better position to know about possible support than our GP. He never mentioned the Alzheimer's Society, he never explained why he had come to the decision he had, and he certainly never mentioned any other possibility than 'pre-senile dementia'.

For a brief while I am told things were better, when the anti-dementia drugs were available to be prescribed. Now that people in the early stages are no longer considered for these drugs, the incentive has gone for regular visits to the consultant. The official advice on services for younger people with dementia is that there should be a named consultant in each area. Clive was referred to a neurologist, but others in similar circumstances end up in the clinics of psychiatrists or geriatricians. There should be someone responsible for liaising with other specialists as required: for example, occupational therapists, speech therapists, community mental health nurses, social workers, genetic counsellors. Oxford still has no named consultant with responsibility for younger onset dementia.

Chapter 4

Dealing with the Diagnosis

It's 5:30 a.m. in autumn – an ungodly time of day, and a horrible day at that. I can hear the rain beating against the window, and my nose tells me it is cold outside the bed-clothes. Clive is just getting up to go swimming – he has done this every day we have been home for the last three years or so. Sundays and bank holidays are included – the swimming pool even opens for 'Early Risers' on Christmas Day. He gets himself dressed in the clothes I laid out last night, says goodbye and goes. I snuggle down under the duvet for another hour. I'm just dozing off when I hear the door open, and Clive comes back. He takes his clothes off and comes back to bed – Brrrr! He's very cold. 'The bike's broken' he announces. I try to find out more, but we both start to get frustrated. That's all he can tell me – the bike is broken, it won't work. When I get up and have time to look, the bike won't work because the front wheel is bent almost in half. I can't imagine how Clive can have managed this and not injured himself, though his anorak is very muddy. I get the cycle carrier out, and drop Clive off at the day centre and his bike at the cycle repair shop.

They are very used to me by now. How the wheel got bent
is something I never discover.

After all the excitement and rushing around to get the succession
of diagnoses, we went home to try and sort out some way of
surviving what was to come. Both OPTIMA and the National
Hospital had been very helpful, advising us about the benefits
available to Clive, and the legal problems we might face, and how
to deal with them. Their advice was:

o apply for Disability Living Allowance

o make wills for both of us, taking particular care to
make good arrangements for looking after Clive and
the children if anything happened to me

o set up an Enduring Power of Attorney for Clive, so
either myself or Clive's brother could legally make
decisions and sign for him

o contact the Alzheimer's Society

o contact our bank to see what they could do to help

o develop a routine for Clive to follow

o make as many contacts as possible of people who
might be helpful as Clive's illness progressed.

We were referred to a geriatricians to see what help might be
available. He was not very helpful. Oxford had an excellent head
injuries unit, to help rehabilitate people who had similar
problems to Clive, though with a different cause. However, as
Clive's illness was progressive, rehabilitation was not an option
and they weren't prepared to consider him. The Adult Mental
Health Team could offer support to people with mental illnesses,
but there was a physical cause for Clive's illness, so they weren't

prepared to consider him. There were some services for the elderly, but Clive was only 45, and it was dubious if they would accept him, or if he would agree to go. In any event, the activities they ran were hardly likely to use up Clive's boundless energy.

About the only concrete advice that came from this session with the geriatricians was about Clive's ability to drive. This was very clear. We had to inform the Driver and Vehicle Licensing Agency (DVLA) and our insurance company. In the meantime, it would be a good idea to ask a local driving school for an assessment of how safe Clive was. Goodbye and good luck.

So we went home and started sorting things out. I wrote to the DVLA and our car insurance company, and arranged an appointment for Clive with a local driving school. The written assessment that came back from the instructor said that, in his opinion, Clive was currently safe to drive, and he recommended a re-test every six months. Given this, the insurance company were prepared to continue to cover him. The DVLA didn't respond for a long time.

We found a friendly solicitor and made our wills. Clive also signed an enduring power of attorney. With the encouragement of the people from OPTIMA, I sent off for the form to apply for Disability Living Allowance, a benefit available then to people under 65 incapable of work. The form that came back was many-paged, and asked the same question several times in a slightly different format. It was mostly aimed at people with a physical disability, and I found filling it in a most frustrating and upsetting experience. It reduced me to tears several times, but I had to persevere, as we needed the money. I posted the form on the last day possible if we were to get the benefit backdated to the day I applied for the form, but the effort paid off – Clive was awarded the allowance at the higher rate.

Our house was owned jointly. The solicitor advised us to transfer ownership to me, and, as Clive was happy to do this, we went ahead. She was right – it saved hassle later on. I also separated our joint bank account, and arranged for Clive's credit card to have a much lower limit. Again, he was in agreement, and I was advised to do so by the National Hospital. They had previously known patients with frontal-lobe dementia (which was their best guess for Clive's illness) who had spent the family savings on a yacht, or an expensive holiday to Australia; as we couldn't afford that I had to do something. I didn't want Clive to be penniless – he had worked hard for his money, and he was entitled to spend it as he wanted to, but unfortunately now I could no longer trust him as I had. Giving him an adequate allowance seemed the best way forward. It was not easy, as the credit card company insisted on increasing his credit limit practically every month, and refused to talk to me about my husband's card, yet I managed. As with many things, I had to.

I contacted the local branch of the Alzheimer's Society, and they sent a very nice lady to see me – a Mrs King. Clive made one of the last jokes I remember him making – he commented that it was a good job her first name wasn't Jo. A typical Clive joke – he had probably been making it since he was five, and that was doubtless why it remained in his memory for so long. I'm assured that it was not the case, but I felt that the meeting started with a query on her part as to who was ill – me or Clive. She put me in touch with two groups of other people whose partner had dementia, and I made it to a few meetings of the nearest group. They were all at least 20 years older than I was; their meetings were in the middle of the day, which meant I had to take time off work, and few of their problems seemed similar to mine. Clive didn't have Alzheimer's disease; his memory was not yet badly affected; he was having difficulty with speech, reading and writing, and the biggest problem was finding ways to occupy him and use the energy that he had used in the past running marathons and jumping out of aeroplanes. It was a sad come-down to being an unemployed, unemployable disabled person.

One of the big discussions at these meetings and in the Alzheimer's Society newsletter was whether to tell the person with dementia about the diagnosis or not. I remembered Clive at a meeting with our GP to discuss the results she had received from the National Hospital. He very forcefully stated that the letter she had in front of her was about him, and therefore he was entitled to read it; he insisted on reading it, and wanted a copy of it for his records. He was certainly not having difficulty with language at that meeting, and Clive being forceful was an intimidating experience. He even banged the desk with his fist. He got a copy of the letter. It made the Alzheimer's Society seem in a different world, with frail, unassuming patients.

We still had to explain things to our children. They were then just coming up to four and five years old, and obviously likely to be aware of odd things happening in the family around them. I discussed it with the nurse at OPTIMA, and she offered to talk to them. So, early one morning, the children, me and the nurse met in the OPTIMA office. None of the other staff had arrived, so we had the place to ourselves, and the nurse had provided croissants and juice. We looked at Clive's scans, and compared them with normal brain scans. There were several plastic models of the brain which could be dismantled and (with difficulty) reassembled. Afterwards the children drew pictures. I don't know how much they understood, or remembered, but we did the best we could to explain things in language they would understand. And I had a tearful interview with the school headmaster to explain the family circumstances.

I bought a phone with programmable memory, and set up the buttons so that Clive could phone his family and friends without needing to remember the number. I got Clive a medic-alert bracelet with an emergency telephone number on it. It was quite a job persuading him to wear it, as he hated any form of jewellery, but we succeeded eventually. We gradually contacted all our friends and Clive's past colleagues. Some remained in touch, and were a great help; some quietly slipped out of our lives, and one or two rang me up to say how sorry they were, but they couldn't stand to see the altered Clive.

We gradually worked out a routine which would keep Clive fit and active, and as independent as possible. Fortunately we had already lived in the current house for a few years, so Clive knew that house and its surroundings quite well. And cycling was his preferred way of travelling about, so he was likely to be able to stay mobile for much longer than if he used a car. The point of a routine is that you don't need to think about it. Making decisions is hard work, and very difficult for people with dementia. The routine reduces the need to make decisions, yet still leaves people with dementia some control over their own lives.

The importance of routine and familiarity was brought home to me a few years ago, when I moved house after five years in one place. Clive and I were moved by the Army every year or so, so I should have been used to it, yet I found the move very disruptive. The light switches were on the wrong side of the door; the stairs had a different layout; it took time to get the washing machine and dishwasher plumbed in, so the routine of washday was lost; all the kitchen cupboards were in different places – you get the idea. It took me a few months to settle into a new routine, and it made me realise how difficult life must have been for Clive.

Clive was a member of the 'Early Risers' swimming club in Abingdon, so every day (including Sunday!) he got up at 5:30 a.m., cycled to Abingdon, swam for an hour and then cycled home, had a bath, and cooked his breakfast of alternately porridge and kipper, with fruit and coffee. Over breakfast, and afterwards as he lingered over his coffee, he read *The Spectator.* He had subscribed to this for decades; he used to read it quickly, then pass it on to me so we could discuss articles. By the time he was diagnosed it took him several days to read it; he would sit with one finger keeping his place and a puzzled and worried frown on his face, yet he kept the subscription going.

Every day he had a fixed activity. On Monday he went to HeadWay: a daygroup run by volunteers for people with head injuries. On Tuesday he cycled into Oxford and saw an acupuncturist. On Wednesday he went to the Abingdon Alzheimer's Club, on Thursday to another group run by volunteers for a mixed group with physical and mental disabilities. On Friday he and I went for a long walk. Saturday was the day for shopping, followed by cinema and pizza with the children, and Sunday was the day for a family outing.

The Abingdon Alzheimer's group was the only group specifically for people with dementia, and Clive was the youngest person who had ever attended; he was very much the same age as the organiser and volunteer helpers. We were all dubious as to whether Clive would fit in and be happy to attend, but the staff were very good. They treated him very much as one of themselves, and tried to find him simple jobs to do. Clive described himself as 'half man, half biscuit', and would say 'I may not be very bright, but I can lift heavy weights'. I think he spent a lot of time moving chairs around the room. They also brought in a yoga teacher once Clive started attending, who was very good at finding exercises that everyone present could do. One of the exercises was, while seated, to lift the feet up and down. The more frail people used to lift their feet a few inches and place them down gingerly; Clive stamped his feet up and down as fast as he could manage. I recently spoke to the staff who worked with him, and realised just how much of a challenge Clive had been to them, and how difficult it had been to work with someone their own age, instead of someone belonging to their parents' generation. The other two day centres Clive attended were aimed at people his age or younger, and he seemed very content to be there.

Our children were then beginning at primary school, and there were fortunately lots of activities not too far away which we could all attend quite happily. I always chose somewhere we could drive to; it was easier and less stressful for me to keep everyone together. When we were at the park or whatever, I felt like a worried mother hen as I tried to keep an eye on everyone, and not lose anyone. We went to swing parks, steam railways, zoos, gardens, museums. Oxford has a beautiful arboretum, and that was a favourite place for picnics in the summer. When the weather was bad we went to the Pitt Rivers Museum to admire the shrunken heads and totem poles. Clive especially loved the steam trains, so we went to Didcot or Quainton quite often. I suppose the steam trains were just being phased out when he was young, which may explain the fascination. Brill Windmill was another favourite place.

I have met many people at conferences and talks who comment on how difficult it must have been to look after someone with dementia and two young children, but I think the age of the children, in fact, made it easier. We could do normal family activities, and Clive could join in. He was not handicapped by not being able to read – the children were only beginning to learn. He could play the chasing games that they all enjoyed, and we soon established that we could all throw a frisbee, but no-one could catch it.

My sympathy goes to those who have a partner with dementia and teenage children. I have no idea how they cope. You will also notice that all our activities cost money, and we got no 'disabled discount' for Clive at any of the places we visited. He wasn't visibly disabled, and I wasn't prepared to spend time arguing. We were very fortunate that we still had money left from Clive's redundancy payout, and my savings from two years in Dubai. Again, my sympathy to those who try to cope with a partner with dementia on a very limited income – I have no idea how they manage either.

A few weeks after Clive's last disastrous outing with the TA, I got a telephone call from his boss. Note that he called me, not Clive. Was Clive going to resign from the TA? I thought about Clive's lifelong service, and said no, I didn't think he was. I rather hoped the Army would be forced to notice Clive's illness – it was, after all, less than a year since his redundancy. A few days later we received a standard letter thanking Clive for his service. I didn't hear from them again until much later. Clive had always told me that the Army looked after its own. So much for that, I thought in my cynical way, and got on with the day-to-day aspects of living.

One of Clive's colleagues had left the Army about the same time Clive did, and very shortly afterwards was diagnosed with aggressive prostate cancer. His wife contacted the Royal British Legion, and was advised to apply for an enhanced pension because of her husband's illness. The cases seemed very similar, so I also wrote to the British Legion. They encouraged my to apply for the same enhanced pension, told me how to get the proper forms, and helped me fill them in – by this stage any additional paperwork reduced me to tears. I received a reply, quite quickly, refusing the pension. I would have given up, but again encouraged by the Legion, I wrote to my MP and asked for an appointment with him to ask for his help. We went to see him one sunny summer day – he was sitting at a desk at the far end of a community hall, and Clive and I walked across the room, and sat down in front of him. I explained the situation. He looked at Clive, and asked how old he was. Clive hesitated, looked at me for help, and then hazarded a guess – 45. 'No', I said to him 'you're 48'. I looked back at the MP. He was white and shaken. He was probably about that age himself. He promised to do what he could, and we left.

We were then asked up for an assessment at the Army hospital in Woolwich. I arranged for someone to look after the children, and off we went. It was a beautiful clear autumn day; we went up to London by coach, crossed London by tube and went out to Woolwich on the train. It was a long journey, probably taking three or four hours. The board seeing Clive was headed by a general. They did a few tests on Clive, and then the General looked at me and explained that there had been a war on, and Clive was just another casualty. It was as close to an apology as Clive was going to get. We came back across London by riverboat – I was rather disappointed that we couldn't manage a trip on a horse and carriage, then we would have managed all forms of transport. Some weeks later Clive was awarded an attributable pension – considerably more than the basic pension we had received. It was backdated until the date we applied for it, not the date Clive left the Army. The Legion wanted me to fight for the further backdating, but I had had enough. It was now two years since Clive's redundancy. He was deteriorating quite fast, and I wanted to spend such time as we had left enjoying our time together, not writing letters and filling in forms.

With hindsight

We were given good advice, we followed it, and it paid off. The enduring power of attorney allowed Clive's brother and me to manage Clive's financial and legal affairs for him when he was no longer capable. Setting up the power of attorney was quite painless; registering it so we could use it was quite traumatic. Not because of the process involved, but because registering it meant we had to formally recognise how much Clive had deteriorated. But had we not had it, the alternative (court of protection) would have been much more traumatic and much more expensive. I was Clive's next of kin, so I also had rights to decide his medical care. In 2007, enduring power of attorney was replaced by lasting power of attorney, which gives the people nominated the right to manage legal, financial and medical matters for someone who is no longer capable.

The benefit Clive received – Disability Living Allowance – is still available, but only for people aged under 65. It is not means-tested, and, although the form I filled in was principally aimed at people with physical disabilities, Clive was given the benefit even though he remained physically fit and active until very late in his illness, so the authorities do recognise dementia. The equivalent benefit for people aged over 65 is Attendance Allowance.

I continued to work, although only by having a very understanding boss, and by working part-time. If you need to give up work to look after a partner with dementia, you can claim Carer's Allowance.

Benefits change. The only advice I can really give to someone with a diagnosis of dementia, or their friend or partner, is to get up-to-date advice and to follow it. Delaying doesn't make it any easier, and does affect the money you will receive, as the benefits cannot be backdated.

I wish I had chased the Army sooner, but I really believed Clive would be given good advice. I was lucky in that eventually I managed to get for Clive the enhanced pension he should have received from the beginning. I meet so many people at conferences, or who call a telephone help line, and one of the first things they mention is redundancy or dismissal. My advice would be not to take no for an answer, but, again, to go to the experts (maybe a trade union, Citizens Advice Bureau or as in my case the Royal British Legion) and follow their advice.

If you or someone close to you thinks they may be in the early stages of dementia, first don't despair. There are other treatable illnesses which cause similar symptoms, and dementia is very uncommon in people under 65 (67 per 100,000). Nag and nag until you get a diagnosis you are satisfied with, and, if you are employed, don't resign and don't accept redundancy.

Chapter 5

Coping with Dementia

'Clive, go sit down.' I'm in the kitchen, getting dinner ready. Raw carrots and peppers for us all. Fish fingers and chips for the children, who are in the sitting room watching telly. Stir-fry for us a bit later. It's hard work, and gets me very annoyed having to cook two meals every day, but Clive and I don't want to live on fish fingers and turkey dinosaurs, and the children won't eat much else. So I do two meals every evening, and everyone else is reasonably happy. Clive is just behind me.

'OK' Clive says cheerfully, and stays put. His illness is progressing, and he doesn't understand much of what is said to him these days. He's also very good at ignoring what he doesn't want to hear. I walk into the sitting room to get bowls for the veg. Clive follows me, and follows me back again. I go back to the sink, and start slicing carrots. Clive hovers about 18 inches away. 'Why don't you go and sit with the children?' I suggest. 'OK' Clive grins, and stays put. I walk round him to turn the oven on, and then out to the garage to get chips and fish fingers from the freezer. Everywhere I go Clive is 18 inches behind me. This is new behaviour. I wonder what's wrong, and I'm beginning to find the constant shadowing a nuisance. Our kitchen is quite small, and Clive is a powerful man. I put a bowl of carrot sticks into his hands, and ask if he can take it through to the children. Maybe he will stay with them and eat. 'OK, anything you say' he agrees, puts the bowl down and watches me. I call one of the children to get the carrots – Rachel comes in, but Clive doesn't follow her out, as I'd hoped he might. Instead, he starts eating the veg I have prepared for the stir-fry. I put fish fingers and chips into the oven to cook. Clive is too close for me to get at the oven comfortably, but he doesn't notice, and I manage. 'The news will be on the TV soon' I say. Clive loves watching the news. 'OK' he says, and stays put. Obviously watching me cook tea is more enthralling than anything else right now.

I move round him to get at the kettle, move round him to get to the sink, and back to plug the kettle in. Into the sitting room to get the teapot and mugs. Back to the kitchen to make tea. All the time Clive is no more than 18 inches away from me. Tea made and poured, I put a mug of tea into his hand. 'Sit down and watch the news' I ask. 'OK' he smiles, puts the tea down and stays put. Time to get the children's dinner out. I move over to the cooker. Clive follows. I get the hot pan out, and move back to close the oven. Clive is too close – I'm worried he will burn himself on the hot pan. I allow a slight edge to enter my voice. 'Clive, go and sit down!' 'OK.' He doesn't move an inch. I manoeuvre round him to get at the plates, dish up the children's dinner, and round Clive again to get at the sink. I take dinner through to the table, and the children settle down to eat. Clive follows me. I move back to the sink and start running hot water to wash up. Clive is even closer now – I can feel his breath on the back of my neck. This is really getting to me now. 'Clive, go and sit down.' 'OK.'

'Clive, please will you go and watch TV?' The 'please' expresses my irritation. I am penned into a corner by Clive. 'OK.' I want to get my own tea and sit down, but Clive is in the way. I use the voice I use to stop the children running into the road. 'Clive, go and sit down.' His face changes. He doesn't smile, or say 'OK'. Instead, he closes in on me and punches me very hard in the ribs, just once. Then he turns and walks out of the house. He is away for an hour or so, and when he comes back he settles to dinner and the news on TV as though nothing has happened. Maybe he has forgotten about it. But I have had a warning I will never forget.

With as good a diagnosis as we could get, most of the essential legal issues sorted out and Clive's routine established, the children and I settled down into a quiet routine of our own. OPTIMA saw Clive every year to see how things were, and six months after each visit they phoned me for a progress report.

Initially, Clive could still drive, and had a reasonable understanding of most of what was said. I worked part-time; I started off on three days per week, and gradually reduced my hours as I had to spend more time with Clive and the children.

To begin with, I got the children ready for school, and then left for work, leaving Clive to take the children to school at a more reasonable hour – school was only a mile away, but it was a narrow country road and not good for walking, so he drove them. Clive had always been very particular about punctuality. We arrived at several parties on the dot of 7:30 p.m., if that was the time we were invited for, to find our hosts in the shower. It took me a long time to persuade him that, while an Army invitation for 7:30 meant 7:29 and 59 seconds, a 'civvy' invitation for 7:30 meant 8:00, or even 8:30. As his ability to tell the time diminished, he became more obsessed with not being late. Eventually a friendly neighbour told me that Clive was leaving the house as soon as I had left, and then school complained that the children were being left outside the locked school gates. So I altered my hours of work, and went to work via school an hour later. It was impossible to communicate to Clive that he should leave later, or that a four-year-old and five-year-old could not be left on their own for 45 minutes until school opened. Clive still picked the children up after school, and they watched TV or played in the garden until I came home and cooked their tea. Then it was bath-time, story-time and bed-time, after which I got dinner ready for Clive and me, and then at last it was gin-and-tonic time.

It may seem extravagant, bad for family relations and frankly rather silly for us to eat separately from the children, and I certainly found it quite onerous, but it worked for us. It started when the children were still toddlers: we had always eaten late, and didn't like having our main meal about 6 p.m. We also like spicy food, which the children wouldn't eat. It saved on family arguments as well; Clive became progressively more obsessive about 'proper eating habits', and wouldn't accept that a four-year-old was unlikely to sit quietly and eat with a knife and fork. So separate mealtimes worked out just fine for us all in the evenings.

Clive had always followed the news and current affairs, seeing it as part of his job, but now he became obsessive. There was news at 6 p.m., news at 7 p.m., news at 9 p.m., news at 10 p.m. and news at 10:30 p.m.. Thank goodness there were no 24-hour news channels then, otherwise the rest of us would have watched no TV at all.

Clive wanted to keep writing, so he kept a diary for me to read when I got in from work, telling me what he had done with the day. I had to work very hard to stop from crying as I read it, with Clive looking on. The language was very flat – first I did…, and then I did…, and then I went…, and then I did… There were lots of crossings-out, where he had taken three or four attempts at a word, and there were many mis-spellings that he had not recognised. It broke my heart, but it was at least another way of communicating with Clive. After a few months the diary was quietly dropped, as Clive found writing it too difficult.

As I said, I programmed a phone with the numbers of Clive's friends and relatives, and my number at work. The phone was a standard model, with a small space next to each button for the name of the person at the other end. Clive used this for a long time, but there came a time when he could no longer decipher the

The hole in the wall ant the Midland bank
was not operating, so I went to [crossed out]
Nat West, I put my card in, but it [crossed out]
It did not give me any mony, [crossed out] that
time the [crossed out] [bank] was open, so
I told one of the staff what had happened.
Then I went to Midland, and told them
They issued me with another card
and then I used it. I have memorised
the number. I got £50, and and I [crossed out] then
[crossed out] saw some of that at Pedal Power
[crossed out] It cost my about a fiver.
Then I got on my bike and went home
At home, I did some [crossed out] hovering

I would now like to tell you what I
did today, today, to I Friday. the When I
got up the first thing I did was to get on
my bike and go swimming. I did my
normal 20 lengths lengthes, and then got
on my bike and went home. Then I had

A page from Clive's diary

names, and he was then unable to make calls independently. I
looked very hard for a different phone with a bigger space next to
the buttons, so I could put a photo there instead of writing the
name, but I couldn't find anything. I told all Clive's relatives, so
they could make a habit of calling him, but of course it wasn't the
same at all. It's a shame, as it seems such a simple idea, and there
must be people other than Clive who would find such a phone
useful.

One of the mistakes I made with the phone was to programme one of the buttons to dial 999. When I set the number up, I was very aware that Clive was often in the house with the children, and I was concerned about someone having an accident. It was a mistake because it meant that there was one button which shouldn't normally be used, and I was expecting a lot of Clive to understand that. I should have removed the number, so that Clive would always contact a friend whichever button he pressed, but I never got round to changing the programme. It was just another item that never made it to the top of the list, and that made me feel guilty.

I was very aware that leaving Clive and the children alone in the house was potentially risky. I wasn't worried about Clive hurting them, but should any disaster happen I was worried that no-one would react appropriately. Apart from major disasters like the house catching fire, or the roof blowing off in a gale, my imagination pictured someone falling down stairs, or pulling a pan of boiling water on top of themselves or sitting in the dark because a fuse had blown, or... One can imagine all sorts of nasty things in the middle of the night. I consoled myself with the thought that no-one smoked, the house had central heating not open fires, the fuses scarcely ever blew, and it would be a major expression of no-confidence in Clive to tell him that I didn't think he was fit to be left in charge of his children. I made sure that the children knew how to use the phone to call for help, and we had discussions (when Clive was out) about when they might call me at work, when they might call 999, and when they might go round to the neighbours for help. I tried to arrange things so that the three of them were only alone in the house for an hour or so. I couldn't arrange things so that I was always there without giving up my job. The whole of that time in our lives was about taking a realistic look at risks and payoffs, and I think I got this balance about right.

Of course, I always had this worry at the back of my mind when I was in the office, and, while I never received one of the nightmare calls, I did get frequent calls from Clive or from one of the day centres he went to, or from someone else connected with Clive. One of my colleagues at work commented later that every time the phone rang at work I turned white, and I think it indicates the stress I was under. I wasn't aware of this at all myself. She also commented that she had never been aware that living with someone with dementia could have such effects, and so in some way she gave me the idea for this book.

Just after we moved house, when I was still trying to pretend that Clive was OK, I was upstairs unpacking. It was a difficult job, as we had moved from a spacious four-bedroom detached house back into a three-bed semi, and I was struggling to find places to put things. Clive and the children were playing downstairs, and eventually I had had enough, so I went down for a cup of tea. There was a lot of noise coming from the sitting room, so I went in to see what was going on. I had left the room fairly tidy, with the big bits of furniture unpacked, and a few boxes against the walls. Clive had started to do some unpacking, but got distracted, and when I opened the door, the three of them were jumping up and, down on the bubble-wrap and throwing balls made from packing paper at each other – they were having a great time. The room was a mess, and I was feeling particularly ratty, so I let loose. 'What do you think you're doing?' I shrieked. 'You're acting like a bunch of five-year-olds.' Then I stopped and looked at them. My daughter was five. My son was four. Clive was in his forties, but, if I was honest, I was beginning to realise he was no longer a 're-sponsible adult'. So I started laughing. Of course they were acting like a bunch of five-year-olds – that was what they were. I always tried to remember that in the future. I joined in the mock fight, and then we had tea and made a game of picking up the bits.

Although that incident happened a year before Clive was diagnosed, it set the pattern for the next few years. I was effec-tively a single parent with three children. The youngsters were growing physically, in individual skills, like reading, writing, and using a knife and fork, and in knowledge and understanding of the world, and Clive was slowly losing those skills and that knowledge. The more I think about it, the more I admire him. It must be terrifying to lose abilities you take for granted – writing a letter, making a telephone call. Even early in his illness, Clive's understanding of what was said was limited. It must have felt like living in China or Japan, where you can't understand what people around you are saying, and yet even more frightening because you know you used to be able to. Yet Clive never showed any despondency, and just kept going, doing his best and trying repeatedly until he got things right.

I was out of the house a lot to begin with, and unfortunately I left before the post arrived in the morning. Clive had always dealt with the family paperwork, and now he filed any letters as soon as they dropped on the mat. It was very frustrating for me, because every evening I had to go and look in all the likely places. To begin with, letters got filed in a reasonable place in the filing cabinet, but that got more and more erratic, and I know there were some letters I never found. We were planning a holiday in Jersey, so I wrote to the local diving club to see if I could join them for some dives. I never got a response, and assumed they had ignored my letter. A few months later, I discovered an invitation to join them, and a list of likely dive sites and contact phone numbers; it had slipped between two files, and was lurking at the bottom of the filing cabinet. I tried to ask Clive just to leave letters out for me to look at, but he never seemed to latch on to the idea.

I was doing a course at work, which was a succession of one-week courses once a month for six months. For the first week, we all had name badges, but they weren't provided afterwards, so I asked if we could be given them for subsequent weeks. On the first day of the third week, we were all issued with name badges again, and I expressed my thanks. When I went home, I removed the badge and left it on my bedside table, then went off to start the evening routine. In the morning, I couldn't find my badge anywhere. I emptied drawers, pulled the bedlinen off the bed, hunted everywhere, but I couldn't find the badge, and eventually I had to go in without it. It caused a lot of hilarity that I had asked for badges, and then not worn my own. I didn't try to explain, but I was fairly certain that I would find it eventually, filed somewhere that had seemed logical to Clive at the time. He became obsessively tidy for quite a while, and it caused me no end of problems.

There was a similar problem with phone calls. If Clive took a message for me, he would try to write it down, but very often I couldn't decipher the message, or who it was from. Asking Clive was a recipe for disaster, as he got very upset. I consoled myself with the thought that most people would try again.

In my youth I used to have a temper, and in fact our families called us 'Hot and Cold', as Clive was so phlegmatic, and I was so fiery. Nowadays I have a reputation for calmness and steadiness. It all came from the years when Clive was ill. I got very good at counting to ten, and then again, and often again. I also changed my priorities. Things that used to seem very important, like matching jacket, skirt and shoes for work, no longer seemed to matter. I learned to go with the flow much more than I ever had.

When Clive was first diagnosed, we were advised to see how fit he was to drive by getting an assessment from a driving instructor. Clive passed the first assessment OK, and so I was happy for him to continue to drive. It meant he could pick the children up from school, and do shopping trips into town. School was a short distance away along a quiet country lane, and the local town was only a few miles away, so I wasn't too concerned. Finally, about six months after the initial assessment, the DVLA responded to my letter, and arranged a driving test for Clive. Unfortunately he failed because he was too cautious, and so I had to act quickly to stop him driving. We were very lucky, because Clive could still get around on his bike, and so losing the licence didn't mean a total loss of independence for him. I think he was rather relieved not to have to drive, but I was commenting one morning that I would have to go via the garage to fill the car with petrol and he offered to do it. I reminded him that he couldn't, and he agreed, but he still went off to look for the car keys.

We had been a two-car family for many years, but that weekend I got rid of both cars, and replaced them with a totally different car – different colour from the others, different make, different style – and always referred to it as my car. Clive accepted the situation, and never tried to drive again.

Clive continued his efforts to help me around the house. I got used to putting the furniture back in the right place after Clive had hoovered, and checking in the airing cupboard that he hadn't put the washing away straight out of the machine. If I allowed the washing to accumulate in the laundry basket, Clive would help by stuffing everything into the washing machine, and washing it all on a very hot wash – he was determined to get everything clean. I soon learned to have a hidden corner for 'hand-wash only' garments – though the number of these diminished as I stopped buying anything that wasn't machine washable, and many items had succumbed to Clive. It was impossible to be cross with him – he was doing his best to help, and I didn't have the heart to try and get him to stop.

He could still do some shopping. I had to be careful not to ask for stuff that was fragile or breakable, as such items didn't travel well in Clive's rucksack, but, as his reading got worse, the things he bought bore less and less relationship to what I had asked for. On one occasion I came home to find the freezer full of ice-cream, and another time he laid in a six-month's supply of fish fingers. Fortunately we weren't trying to live on a tight budget – that would have been impossible without keeping Clive penniless.

Clive had two cockatiels as pets. Again, he had asked for my approval before getting them, and by this time they were a few years old – about as old as our daughter. They were friendly enough, though they made a tremendous mess, dropping birdseed in their cage and then flapping their wings to spread the mess through the house. Clive used to let them out every evening, and they would come and sit on our shoulders. Clive developed an obsession about their food. Practically every time he went shopping, he would come home with another packet of birdseed, until the cupboard where we kept it was full. One of the packets must have been infested, because the room, and then the house, was invaded by some sort of moth. I eventually tracked down the source, but it took forever to get rid of the moths. Clive promptly started filling the cupboard again.

We had a rabbit jelly mould, and Clive loved making a jelly for tea. The children's favourite flavour was raspberry. If time was short, Clive used to put the jelly mixture in the freezer to speed up the cooling process. The freezer was in a corner of the dining room, across a pale green carpet from the kitchen. The mixture more than once landed up on the carpet, making a horrible mess for me to find when I came in from work. Again, it was impossible to be cross, but I had to count to ten several times. Jelly mixture is very sticky stuff to get out of a carpet. Although Clive always tried to clean things up, all he managed to do was spread the mixture further.

When there was a suggestion that Clive might go to the Abingdon Alzheimer's Club, I went with him to meet the staff, and have a look round. For some reason, Clive refused to come with me in the car, so he went on his bike and I drove. By some miracle we met outside the centre – I had managed to get through to Clive where to go. He leant his bicycle against the cycle rack, and draped the lock around the saddle. We were in the middle of town, and I was feeling rather poor, so I pointed out to Clive that the lock wasn't actually doing anything. He disagreed, and began to get cross. I insisted that he lock the bike properly, and pulled the lock off the saddle. Clive didn't say a word; he just grabbed the lock off me, pulled the bike past me, got on and cycled off in a temper. That was when I learned that it wasn't worth the effort of trying to talk Clive out of anything he wanted to do, or into anything he didn't want to do. I had to write to all the people he saw regularly, to tell them. As his understanding of language and his memory got worse, it became more of a problem. Anything he wanted to do had to be done immediately; presumably he was worried he would forget. But it got increasingly dangerous to get in his way. You could sometimes distract him, but not very often.

Clive and I were used to non-verbal communication, as we had been diving buddies for a long time, and it is impossible to talk underwater, so divers communicate with hand-signals. This helped a little in the early stages, but the sort of signals divers use are very simple – OK, not OK, look over there, come over here... Clive tended to nod and smile whether he had understood or not. I was reminded of the time when I was one of a group of English computer people employed by a German consultancy. We all took intensive lessons in German, and after a few months we went out with our partners and some German colleagues for lunch. The conversation was in German, and I at least was nodding and smiling, and catching about half of what was said. Everything was hunky dory until one of the English partners asked us to translate, and there was an embarrassed silence. We were all fairly sure of the gist of what was being said, but no-one was prepared to commit themselves to a translation. Clive must have felt like that: always on the edge of understanding, but never being quite sure.

It was difficult to find activities for Clive and the children to enjoy together. When we were outside, it was fine. We could play ball games, or go to the swings, or just run around; one summer we flew kites a lot, and we went swimming almost every week. But, as winter came on, we couldn't spend so much time outdoors. I bought some soft indoor balls, and a twister set. We had a mini-trampoline, and a loop-the-loop car set, but the favourite game developed from Twister and the mock fights they had always enjoyed, and was just a general free-for-all, with tickling and gentle hits given and received by all. As the children got bigger, and Clive's understanding of his strength got less, I worried about someone getting hurt. At the same time, I didn't want to stop what eventually was Clive's only way of interacting with his children. So we developed a modification: if at any time anybody said 'Stop', the game had to stop immediately. This seemed to work very well, and the game continued until Clive had to leave us.

The one job that Clive continued to be able to do almost to the end was to mow the lawn. He started by mowing the grass and leaving the flower beds alone, but next summer he mowed the flower beds as well. Eventually I had to set the mower up, and one day I found him lifting the mower up in the air to drop it onto some of the shrubs in the garden. I rushed out to remonstrate, and for a few weeks the shrubs were protected by multicoloured ribbons tied around them, but even they proved ineffective. Clive had never been a keen gardener, and it seemed to me he was getting revenge for all the weeding I had asked him to do in the past. I grew all my flowers in pots after that, and they were safe from Clive.

With hindsight

'How did I survive?' I'm often asked, and I have to smile. Stop the world, I want to get off! I had to survive: I had no choice. The alternatives were intolerable – foster carers for the children, nursing home or mental hospital for Clive. More to the point is how I found the strength to survive. I always managed to get to the gym two or three times a week, which certainly helped. The gym was just across the road from the office, so I could pop in at lunchtime. I learned not to think of the big picture, but just of small things that I could achieve in the time I had. For about two years, my definition of a successful day was one where the children's lunch boxes were washed ready for the morrow before I went to bed. Lots of things that had been important to me went by the board. We stopped entertaining. My housekeeping, which was never very good, became worse. Ironing was something other people did. I went to work in jeans and T-shirt. The car never got washed. But no-one ever got food poisoning, and the car, while very grubby, never ran out of petrol or broke down.

Understanding why Clive acted the way he did helped. There were many things I could have done more quickly and easily on my own, but I tried to allow Clive to do what he could, and develop coping strategies for when things went wrong. It seemed very important for him that there were things he could still contribute to family life. I got very good at counting to ten, at looking the other way, at not interfering. But some things, like the times when Clive followed me around, I found very difficult to live with. I knew why he was following – he needed the reassurance of having me in sight. It broke my heart to think of my strong, independent husband being reduced to such a state. But, despite that, it took all my efforts not to shout, and push him away. Knowing the cause didn't make such behaviour tolerable.

I started by having lists of jobs to do, but I soon stopped, because I found it too depressing. The lists never got any shorter, but just grew and grew. The things that needed doing were obvious: a foul smell when I opened the fridge indicated that something was lurking at the back growing mould; a sticky patch on the carpet suggested that Clive had spilled some jelly mix; wails from the children meant that I needed to do some washing or some shopping. My motto became 'never do today what you can put off till tomorrow'. It worked pretty well. If I managed to put the job off indefinitely, it was obviously not that important. Important things to me were creating an environment where Clive could keep going, looking after the children, and trying to keep some time and brain power free for work. People used to ask me what I did 'for myself', but I actively avoided having any time on my own, because I had forgotten all the things I used to be able to do. My luxury was time in the gym, where I concentrated on counting. When I had any free time, I used to play computer patience. It was never something I particularly enjoyed, but it was a sort of mental anaesthetic. The one thing I didn't want was time to think about the future.

Chapter 6

Sinking

Clive and I are at Hyde Park Corner, waiting for the bus back to Oxford. We're on our way back home after a few days away on our own. Only a few minutes more until the bus is due. Clive hasn't much speech left by now, but he is jiggling up and down, and I wonder if he needs the loo. Fortunately the bus has just fitted loos, so we should be OK. I smile at Clive, then turn away to look down the road for the bus. When I turn back, Clive has gone. I look around, and can just see him dashing down the underpass towards Marble Arch tube station. I call his name, but he doesn't stop. Problem. We have two rucksacks and a plastic bag with presents for the children. By the time I have collected these and set out in pursuit, Clive is out of sight. I don't know what to do. I go back to the bus stop to consider. At least Clive is still safe in traffic. I look around, but there is no helpful policeman in sight. I don't have a mobile phone – they are still very big and very expensive. It seems to me the best thing I can do is wait for a while, and hope he can find his way back to me. Unfortunately the subway system at Marble Arch is pretty extensive, with several exits, but I can't think of much else to do. I mentally rehearse a conversation with anyone I might ask for help – bus driver, tour guide, friendly passer-by. The mind boggles. I decide to give him half an hour before doing anything. Just as the time is up, he appears, and gives me a friendly smile and a big hug. The bus turns up and we go home. Another interesting outing with Clive is survived.

We managed all together at home for quite a long time. Things settled down into a routine for us as well as for Clive. School Monday to Friday. Shopping Saturday morning (how I got to hate that supermarket), and often out to the cinema and then for a pizza in the evening; out for a walk or to some farm or museum on Sunday. It wasn't great, but no-one complained too loudly, and we didn't have many dramas. Then in April 1996 I fell pregnant again. I knew it was going to be very difficult managing with a new baby in the house, but nevertheless I was overjoyed. I told everybody, and started making plans for how we could manage. I talked to some of the day centres Clive went to about the possibility of him staying overnight from time to time, or maybe going for longer hours, or at weekends. I told my colleagues at work, and we all went out to lunch to celebrate. I told the family, my mother and Clive's family. Everyone looked dubious; no-one said anything except 'Congratulations'. I got to 12 weeks, and then I miscarried.

Nothing had changed, really. Clive still kept to his routine. The children and I still went down to the river to feed the ducks, out to the cinema, out for a pizza… When school started again I packed lunch boxes, washed shirts, delivered children to school and waited at the school gate in the afternoon. We still watched children's TV, then the news at 6 p.m., 7 p.m., 9 p.m. and 10 p.m. Yet everything had changed for me. I no longer felt I could cope with the world. I signed off sick – I was totally incapable of thinking straight. I had always trusted my body, and now it had let me down. I mourned for my lost child, for my vanishing husband and for my vanished invincibility.

Of course life went on. After a few weeks I went back to work; I couldn't work as well as I used to be able to, but there were a lot of routine things I could still do OK. I started staying up later than Clive, pretending to work but actually playing patience, so that he would be asleep before I came to bed. We had always made love in the morning, but Clive was starting to get amorous in the evening as well, and I didn't feel I could cope. My mantra from this time was 'just keep putting one foot in front of the other', and that's what I did.

In October it was Clive's birthday, and I wanted him to enjoy it, so I asked what he wanted for a birthday present. I already knew that answer, as he had been to a show in London with some Army friends earlier, and was continually looking at the programme and telling me what a good time he had had. I had also planned my response – I was going to ask one of the same friends to take Clive out for the evening. But many of them were away, and I chickened out of asking the rest, so I borrowed the programme to get the address. Clive and I had been to cabarets in Paris, Amsterdam and Berlin, and I was hoping for something similar, but it was not to be. It was a strip show, pure and simple. No singers, no comics, no magicians; nothing other cabaret shows had had. An exclusively male (apart from me) middle-aged audience and a succession of very slim, athletic naked girls on the stage. Clive enjoyed the show, and didn't seem to think it at all strange that I was there with him. I tried not to show my embarrassment, and after the show took Clive to a restaurant for dinner. Clive certainly enjoyed his evening out, and it was something of an education for me.

Shortly afterwards we heard some really excellent news – the Army had awarded Clive a enhanced pension because of his illness. They still wouldn't accept that he had been ill while in service, and so the pension wasn't backdated, but it did mean a considerable increase in our income from then on. I felt I could afford to spend some money, and decided it was time to fulfil a rash promise to take the children (and Clive, of course) to Florida and Disneyland.

Clive was by now having real difficulties with normal activities, so I consulted widely before we went. No-one actually told us not to go, though there were many worried looks. I knew I couldn't manage on my own, so I persuaded a diving friend to come with us. I wanted to avoid the crowds, so I arranged to take the children out of school, and we went at the beginning of January. I roped in more friends to take Clive and the children out for the day while I packed, and then to deliver us to the airport and see us through check-in. We nearly came unstuck at the first hurdle, when Clive dashed out of the car and off in search of a toilet at the wrong terminal in Gatwick, but we retrieved him, and got onto the plane. Our bags were waiting for us in Florida, as was my diving friend and a hire car. I had booked a self-catering villa (restaurants were no longer comfortable places for any of us) a few miles from Disneyland.

Apart from the temperature, Florida was everything I had hoped. It was really cold, but the sun shone, and we enjoyed the theme parks (I developed a real taste for roller coasters), snorkelled with manatees (that really was cold, but still a memorable experience) and had the great luck to see the space shuttle take off. We went to see *Toy Story* before it was out in England, which made the children very happy, and, all in all, it was a great trip. We all enjoyed it, and I'm very glad we went when we did. We couldn't have gone very much later in Clive's illness, as it would have been impossible for us both to manage the travelling and all the changes in routine. Many people thought I was mad to try and take Clive so far from home – to anyone in a similar position my advice would always be to go for it.

The Christmas festivities followed by two weeks in America did nothing for my waistline, and so a few weeks later I decided to get a bit of exercise, and join my neighbour at the local badminton club. The club met quite late on Sunday evening, so I got the children in bed, settled Clive in front of the TV news, and went off to Abingdon. Fortunately my neighbour drove. I warmed up very carefully, and joined in a game. After a few minutes, I fell over. It felt as though someone from an adjacent court had run into me and trodden on the back of my heel, so I waited for the apologies, and the 'are you alright?' But there was silence. After a few minutes my partner asked if I was going to get up and continue, and I realised I couldn't control my right foot. When I lifted my leg, the foot flopped up and down uncontrollably and rather uncomfortably. The sports centre staff came over with a first aid kit, and then went off to phone for an ambulance. I had broken my Achilles tendon. At the hospital I was plastered up from toe to hip, with my toes pointing downwards like a ballet dancer, given a pair of crutches, helped into a taxi, and told to report tomorrow morning for treatment.

I got home about 1 a.m., and found getting into the house very difficult. There was a step of about six inches at the door, and nothing steady to hold on to. I tried to balance on my good leg and ease my pointed toes over the threshold, but couldn't manage. Eventually I sat down and inched in backwards on my backside. When I turned round I found Rachel asleep in a corner of the kitchen under her duvet. I hadn't telephoned to say where I was, as I assumed everyone would be asleep, but Rachel had tried to stay awake until I came home. When I didn't turn up at the appointed time, she had got her duvet and camped out by the door. We had a good cuddle, and I had a bit of a cry, then she helped me upstairs (backwards on my bum again) to bed.

I can't remember much about the next few days. My neighbour took me to hospital to be properly plastered (very much the same format), which they would keep me in for a month, then change the cast to gradually bring my foot back to the normal right-angled position. I don't know how or if the children got to school that day – probably the neighbour took them, as they were too young to leave at home on their own. Clive did his own thing as he always did. That evening the neighbour and I got plastered on gin-and-tonics. I made several desperate telephone calls to Social Services, who said they were working on things. Of course, I rang my mother, who agreed to come down and help out. The local Alzheimer's Society branch helped with shopping, and paid for a taxi service to get the children to and from school. My mother arrived from Yorkshire, but she had done lots of gardening and clearing out of the garage before she set out, and on the journey her sometimes dodgy back had become very painful, and she had a very bad dose of sciatica. I cooked a shoulder of lamb for dinner, but neither of us could carry it to the table. I couldn't get Clive to understand what was wanted, and I thought the children were far too young to carry something so hot and heavy. I put the dish on the floor and crawled along behind it pushing it in front of me. It was Thursday evening.

The next day I again rang Social Services. They seemed to think that, as my mother had arrived, we didn't need any further help. In fact, although her being there was a great comfort, she needed as much looking after as any of us. Clive did his best, but really didn't understand what was going on. He could still make a cup of tea, but he would leave mine on the table out of reach, and then be upset because I didn't drink it. He could see me moving around, and I couldn't get through to him that I couldn't carry anything while I was using crutches.

Saturday was Rachel's birthday. I hadn't been able to get her a present, or a birthday cake, or do anything to celebrate. It was her eighth birthday, and she was very upset. In desperation, I phoned the wife of one of Clive's colleagues, and she organised someone to come round and take the children out for the day.

Gradually things were sorted out. The chairman of the local Alzheimer's carer's group turned up reliably and consistently to take me for my hospital appointments. Friends and neighbours helped with shopping, until Social Services finally sprang into action, and sent someone for two hours once a week to take me shopping. My mother's sciatica improved. Clive continued to do his own thing, but happily without any need for more assistance than before. When the Easter holidays arrived, my sister-in-law came across to take the children to stay with her. My mother decided to move closer to me; her house in Yorkshire was getting too big for her to manage. Much as she loved the acre of garden, she found she was no longer capable of looking after it the way she wanted to. I had never thought she would leave Yorkshire, but I was delighted that she would be close by. She had been an English teacher, and Oxford offered easy access to more theatres and evening classes than were available in a small Yorkshire village. So, while the children were at school and Clive off at day centres, we went off house-hunting, me with my leg in plaster. Mum went back to Yorkshire to sort her house out; my Achilles tendon knitted itself back together again, and life got back to normal – normal for us.

At Christmas, I had promised Clive a trip to Paris. We had been to Paris a few times earlier, and wouldn't have the opportunity for many more trips. Clive couldn't understand my broken leg, and kept nagging about this trip I had promised. So, as soon as I was mobile again, I booked us Eurostar tickets and a hotel in Montmartre. It was probably June by this time, and it was glorious sunny weather, not too hot.

We nearly came unstuck in London. There were roadworks in Oxford, and the London coach had taken much longer than I had allowed, so we ended up rushing across London by tube to try and catch our train. Clive was never good when the routine was broken, and he was beginning to have real difficulty understanding anything new. He found London very unsettling, and stayed very close to me. The tube had just installed automatic barriers which were a surprise to both of us. You shoved your ticket in a slot, and the barrier let one person through. Clive wasn't prepared to be separated from me by even a few inches, and fortunately we both stayed on the outside of the barrier. I don't like to think about what Clive's reaction might have been if we had in fact been separated. As it was, I was separated from my ticket, and with Clive behind me like a siamese twin, I had to find a manned entrance, explain the problem, and get us through together. This took some time, as Clive still looked very healthy and normal, and the guard was suspicious I was pulling his leg. We made it to Waterloo with about two minutes to spare, and settled into our seats.

Clive had followed the progress (and non-progress) of the Channel Tunnel with great interest as it was built, and the year before, when we were planning this trip, he had looked forward to taking the train under the Channel, but I am sure he had no understanding whatsoever of where we were. I found crossing the Channel by Eurostar both very impressive and totally boring – it was just a normal train journey, only dark for some of it. Clive didn't seem to notice anything.

Paris was a bit scary. My French was never very good – I was much more fluent in German. Clive had always been the French interpreter, only he wasn't any longer. After the fun in London, I wasn't prepared to risk the Metro, and I have never been very good at finding taxis. So we walked everywhere. Fortunately our hotel was quite central, and the weather was really nice.

We had dinner on the roof of the Pompidou Centre, lunch just off the Champs Elysées and picnics by the Seine. We visited the Eiffel Tower, going up by the lift and down by the stairs. We went on a *bateau mouche*. We went to see the shows at the Lido, the Crazy Horse and the Moulin Rouge. It was expensive, but I didn't care. We walked for miles, and my Achilles tendon developed a lump the size of a pigeon's egg. We got on the train home with rucksacks clinking with French wine and presents for everyone at home. It had been a great trip, but I had found it very wearing having to make all the decisions myself. I was used to a democracy, and being able to share ideas with Clive. It felt very wrong not being able to ask him what he would like to do – much worse than when we were at home.

Clive was having more difficulties with everyday living. He could still cook his own breakfast and make a cup of tea or coffee, but he was having difficulty with lunch. Ever since the children were small he had been able to cook lunch, always cheese on toast or coddled eggs. A friend had given him some egg coddlers, and he took great pleasure in making eggs to suit everyone – Tabasco in mine, Worcester sauce in his, and a pinch of salt each for the children. He forgot who liked what, and then he forgot how to break eggs into the coddlers, and then how to boil them. I tried not to watch, and to help by laying things out in the right order in the kitchen. He tried to cook cheese on toast, but forgot the toast, and just laid the slices of cheese in the grill pan and cooked them. It made a dreadful mess, and it broke my heart to see the look of puzzlement on his face.

He started finding it difficult to dress himself. I had to put his clothes out on his chair in the right way: socks, trousers, shirt, vest and underpants. He would button the shirt wrongly, or not at all. Sometimes the vest would go on back to front. If he knocked the pile of clothes onto the floor, the vest would go on last. He had always been very particular about clean clothes, but now I had to make sure to remove dirty clothes to the laundry basket. I started getting telephone calls from the swimming pool attendant – an incredibly kind, understanding fellow. 'Helen, Clive took someone else's jumper home today – can I drop round and collect it please?' Clive could still manage to cycle to the pool, change, swim, get dressed again and cycle home, but sometimes he found the wrong pile of clothes. On one occasion the pool was closed for maintenance, but while they had locked the door to the changing rooms, the door to the pool was open. Clive just swam in his clothes and came home wet.

He paid for things mostly by credit card, but occasionally (maybe to buy a cup of coffee) he paid cash. He started not being able to manage the loose change, and would just take a handful of coins from his pocket and proffer it to allow the waiter or shop attendant to help themselves. Fortunately he was still a big strong man, so I had few worries about him being mugged in the street. Thank goodness this was in the days before chip and pin, which would have defeated Clive entirely by this stage. He could manage a scrawl in the right box on the credit card slip, and it was rarely refused.

He started getting lost on his way to various places. He would set out for a day centre at the usual time, and a few hours later I would get a phone call. 'Helen, is Clive coming today?' Normally he found his way there eventually; I think he did many circuits of the Oxford ring road. I never found out where he had been, and I tried not to worry. It seemed better for him to get lost occasionally than for me to try and stop him setting out. Some people bugged me. 'Helen, you really ought to stop Clive…[cycling/ swimming/shopping or whatever].' There was never an explanation of *how* I should stop Clive, who was five foot ten and 13 stone, from doing anything he wanted to. I'm five foot two, and used to be 7 stone. And there was the question of what he did instead. I tried to make sure he was unlikely to hurt anyone else – his cycle was covered with reflectors and lights, and Clive himself resembled a Christmas tree. And I did act very quickly to stop him driving when the DVLA decided he was not fit to drive.

I had to write to all the day centres he attended, and make clear that I did not hold them responsible for Clive's safety, and to make sure that they understood that if he wanted to do something and could not be distracted they must not try to stop him. Clive was normally very happy and easy to 'manage' (horrible thought), but if he wanted to do something, he naturally wanted to do it immediately before he forgot. That was about the only time when he could be physically difficult. If he wanted to achieve some end and you were stopping him, he would do his best to get round you, but, if you persisted, he would go over you, and he had been an Army officer for all of his working life. One of the day centres was close to a big supermarket, and Clive liked to wander round there. Alas, there was a busy road between the two. Clive adopted the 'cars bounce off me' attitude of his parachuting days; it was scary to watch, but he was always OK.

We went to stay with his sister for a few days, and made sure there was a bike for Clive to use, and that he could find his way to the local swimming pool. Fortunately they also had an Early Riser session. Clive set off for his swim, but came home minus shoes and socks. He had managed to find the rest of his clothes, but not those items. He had cycled home (about five miles) in bare feet in October. I drove him back, and we managed to find the shoes and socks underneath a chair in the café. That was Clive all over. Little things like losing shoes and socks would not stop him doing things.

He started forgetting when he had had a bath. He always had a bath after swimming and before breakfast; now he very often had another bath after breakfast. Initially this caused problems, as we ran out of hot water. I had the water heating on morning and evening only, to save money. However after many complaints I realised I could not always distract Clive, and it seemed unfair to make him bath in cold water, so I changed the heating. On occasions he had four baths a day – better than no baths in four days, I told myself.

He also stopped using a safety razor. Ever since I had known him, Clive had shaved wet. He often shaved twice a day, as he hated any suggestion of a five o'clock shadow. He tried to grow a beard on one skiing holiday, but I found the stubble far too uncomfortable on my sunburn when I kissed him, and asked him to shave it off. Apart from that time, he had been always been clean-shaven. He found the wet shaving too much to manage, so started using an electric razor. Alas, when he cleaned it out, more often than not he lost the foil, and came to me with a plaintive 'Helen, it's not working'. I don't know what the man in the shop thought – I came in for a spare foil at least once a week.

He gradually extended the area he shaved – the sideburns got shorter and shorter, and he started shaving round the back of his neck. Eventually he had a mop of black hair at the very top of his head, and was clean-shaven everywhere else, like the reverse of a monk's tonsure. I was quite amused when I heard some passers-by discussing his highly fashionable hair style. I learned not to say anything, as I had when clothes went on in the wrong order, or shirt buttons didn't come out right. It was much more important to me to keep Clive happy and confident, as much as that was possible.

He stopped even pretending to read. When he started to become ill, I noticed he had stopped reading books, but he had persisted with *The Spectator*, albeit reading very slowly, with his forefinger glued to the page to keep his place. And then even that stopped, and the envelope didn't get opened when it dropped on the mat. I cancelled the subscription, and have never opened another copy. Maybe one day. I still have the last book I can remember him reading. It is *A Distant Mirror*, Barbara Tuckman's history of the Black Death. Despite Clive's recommendation, I have never succeeded in reading it. Again, maybe one day.

One of my friends, whose husband had fronto-temporal dementia, told me how her husband sat for hours each day reading a dictionary: trying to relearn the words he was forgetting. We were both in tears.

My GP and Social Services finally twigged the stress the whole family was under, and started a series of review meetings. We met once a month – with my GP, a teacher from school, Clive's social worker and Clive's consultant – and reviewed the situation, and mostly they decided that they couldn't do much to help. I kept quiet about how bad things were. I don't know if it was a sensible fear or not (and I was at that time in no fit state to judge), but I was very worried that the 'official mind' might think that an appropriate response was to remove the children, and place them in foster care. It was, after all, a time when families in Sheffield and Scotland were broken up by Social Services on the unfounded suspicion that the children were being abused. The principal feeling I got from these meetings was a confirmation that we were on our own; no-one could think of any help that would be acceptable to Clive. I often came away wishing that they would cancel the meetings and give me the money saved; at least I could then invest in days out or tasty ready-cooked meals.

Oxfordshire started a 'relief to carers' scheme, and I applied for help, but initially I was refused on the grounds that 'I was asking for help a babysitter could provide'. I may have been, but it was actually almost impossible to get a babysitter that Clive would allow in the house. I did try to get some outside help from the various caring agencies, but it was never actually very helpful. I asked one agency to provide someone to collect the children from school, bring them home and cook their tea, so I could stay at work until a reasonable hour. The first person they provided was a non-driver; the second had a car with no rear seat belts. I could live with that, and happily signed a piece of paper saying so, but the driver was not so happy, and I continued to leave work at 3 p.m. every day. My boss was amazingly tolerant.

It was very difficult finding a babysitter to look after the children, so that I could have some time to myself. I eventually found a wonderful lady who was unfazed by Clive's sometimes bizarre behaviour, and a great support to me and the children. One weekend before I broke my leg, I arranged for her to come for the day so that I could go diving. I had to leave before she arrived; I needed the early start in order to catch the tide. As I was driving past Winchester, the mobile phone rang. It was the babysitter. She had turned up and Clive had sent her away as she wasn't needed, as he was there to look after his children. What was she to do? I told her to go away. If Clive didn't want her there, she could hardly stay in the house. And I turned round at the next exit, and went home. After that, I gave up attempts to get away for the day.

Many of the problems with the outside world came because Clive looked absolutely normal. If you spoke to him, he might not have understood more than one word in three, but he would nod and smile very convincingly. Occasionally he would recognise a phrase, or a single word, which would be enough to trigger an anecdote. If you spent much time with Clive, you realised that these anecdotes came out as if from a tape recorder;

the words, the phrasing and the intonation never varied. But, if you only heard an anecdote once, it sounded very convincing. Visitors to the day centres Clive attended often assumed he was one of the staff.

Clive gave up going to acupuncture. He had been going for a long time, and he seemed to be very happy to continue. It was something he had organised himself in the very early days of his illness, possibly even before we got a diagnosis, and he made the appointments himself, got himself there and back again, and managed the payments. He even succeeded in finding the new surgery when the doctor he saw moved. However, there was a very unpleasant episode when he accidentally took someone else's coat. When I found out, I got the coat back to them as soon as possible, but they still asked Clive to stop coming. There seemed to be a feeling that he had taken the coat deliberately. It was a shame, and brought home to him how his illness was progressing. And it was a break in the routine, and another afternoon when he was home on his own with no activity organised.

It was becoming very clear that the family needed a break from looking after Clive. I spent so much time fixing things – the bike, the shaver, sorting out endless mix-ups – that I didn't have any time to spare to spend with the children. So it was arranged for Clive to spend a weekend in the local psychiatric hospital. It was sold to Clive as him 'needing to go in for some tests', and so rather reluctantly he agreed. I took him in one Friday morning. I found it a grim place – an old Victorian building, with long wards with some very distressed people in. We had a good weekend, not doing anything special, just mooching around, watching TV and chatting. When I picked Clive up on Monday morning, he was in a filthy mood. There hadn't been any tests; no-one had wanted to see him, and he had been ignored all the time he was there. You understand this was Clive's take on things – I am sure it was not so bad, but he felt he was being messed around by the system, and had missed some of the remaining time he had with his family. We never tried that again.

The next attempt was for Clive to go and stay with his mother. But, again, he was out of his own environment, and I think she found him very difficult to keep entertained. She lived next to a very busy road, and worried a lot about Clive having an accident. I sympathised, and was not surprised when she said a repeat visit was not on.

A few weeks later we tried another approach. I booked a weekend away in Ironbridge (we stayed at the Tontine Hotel. A tontine was an early investment scheme in which the survivor took the lot, so the name appealed to my ghoulish sense of humour, and Social Services arranged for someone to come to the house at mealtimes to prepare Clive's food. I can't remember how I got away. Maybe I chickened out, and left while Clive was out, but that seems unlikely. However, it would have been very difficult to explain to him that we were going away for the weekend and not taking him with us. Why should we want to leave him out of a family outing?

Anyway, we had a great time in Ironbridge, and we came home on Sunday evening to find that Clive and the house were still in one piece. He couldn't tell me how things had been, but we were all happy to be back together again. Nonetheless, it was not an experience we repeated. I felt we had been lucky, and didn't feel sufficiently desperate to gamble again.

The last attempt was very successful. One of the OPTIMA nurses had been to a conference, and heard another nurse speak about the care home she was involved with. It did not cater to people with Alzheimer's but for adults with behavioural problems. It was very small – it only had four or five people staying at any time – and aimed to provide lots of physical activity. We visited; Clive seemed to like the place and agreed to come and stay 'for a holiday'. He stayed for two weeks. It was the summer holidays, and the children were home, but, instead of taking advantage of Clive's absence to enjoy our time together, I felt I needed to work, and so they went away for a week to one of the 'adventure camps' available. It was a disaster. They were unhappy there, and I was desperately unhappy at home on my own. I did manage to force myself to finish off a work project, but it was no fun. I never made that mistake again. When I picked the children up, we all agreed that we functioned better as a threesome than individually. And no more 'adventure camps'.

Steve had been one of Clive's colleagues, and had settled fairly close to us when he left the Army – the Abingdon area was central to several Army bases, and quite a few colleagues bought houses in the area. He had kept in touch with Clive, and sometimes took him out to lunch, or to a pub in the evening. He could see how things were, and managed to organise a rota of people who had known Clive. Someone came every Saturday morning, took Clive out for a walk, or some sort of outing, and returned him at tea-time. This was a godsend. It gave me time with the children, and it gave Clive time with his Army friends. Many thanks to Steve, and to everyone involved.

I finally managed to get a blue disabled parking badge for Clive. I had been refused earlier, because Clive could walk for miles, but at last I was advised by someone who knew the system and could convince others just how disabled Clive in fact was. It made my life much easier, being able to park close to the shops and day centres.

One of the day centres Clive used to go to was a long way from home, several miles away and almost the other side of Oxford. Clive had more and more difficulty finding his way there, and sometimes only just got there in time to turn round and come home. The staff were very worried by this (I was much more fatalistic than they were), and they arranged for the centre's transport to pick Clive up. This was all talked through with Clive, but I don't think he actually understood any of it. When the minibus arrived in the morning, he sat on the sofa and refused to go. 'If I can't get there on my own, then I'm not going.' He could not be talked out of it, and that was the end of that day centre as far as he was concerned.

We were all concerned about Clive's growing inability to find his way to places he used to know. He always found the way home, but sometimes he could be away for hours, and no-one had any idea where he was. One of the OPTIMA nurses mentioned a friend who was researching the use of radio tags to trace people who might get lost. It sounded a good idea, and I contacted him. He had to check that the tag was compatible with Clive's pacemaker, but no-one could think of any reason why they should upset each other, and so I agreed to give it a try. The tracking device was about the size of a pack of cards, and after much discussion we attached it to Clive's belt. I never used it to find Clive, but I had to track the device a few times, after Clive left it behind. I felt a right idiot, up on a hill just outside Abingdon, and close to the main Oxford–Abingdon road, waving the tracker about. It was like a TV aerial, and about 50 centimetres long. I successfully tracked the belt to the local sports centre, and had to send someone else in to retrieve it from the men's changing rooms. Still, it made me feel a lot happier that I had a chance of finding Clive if he did get lost.

Christmas came and went. Another disaster struck: our kind, reliable, not particularly elderly babysitter died suddenly and unexpectedly on Christmas Eve of a heart attack. I didn't find out in time to get to the funeral – she had lived alone, and, when she didn't answer the phone, I assumed she had gone to visit some friends for Christmas. I only found out when her neighbour rang, having found my phone number in her address book.

Clive had attended a day centre run by volunteers for people with head injuries. The people who ran it were very kind and competent, but they started to express worries about how well they could look after Clive, and eventually refused to continue taking him. The only day centre he continued going to was the Alzheimer's Club in Abingdon, and they managed to give him an extra day.

It was winter by now, and cold, dark and miserable in the mornings. Clive found the cycle to the pool more and more difficult, and eventually the lifesaver, who was by now a good friend of us all, arranged to pick Clive up. I was worried he would again refuse to go, but John managed to talk him into it, and for the next few months drove well out of his way every day to take Clive swimming, and then return him.

Clive went to the respite home for another two weeks. The local Alzheimer's branch had paid for the first session; this time I had to pick up the tab, but it seemed well worth the £800 or so it cost. Clive was not so happy this time. The weather was worse, and I think they managed fewer outdoor activities, but he was still prepared to keep going, so I booked a session for the Easter holidays. No activity holidays for the children this time – we would just mooch round at home. That felt like a real luxury to me. By this stage I very much felt that the house belonged to Clive, and the rest of us had to fit in around him.

One very wet weekend, we did our usual Saturday activities – shopping in the morning, trip to Oxford in the afternoon, visit to the cinema (we saw *Jumanji* and I was more scared than anyone else) and home via the pizza parlour. When we got home, I was all ready to start on the bath-story-bed routine, but Clive felt the need for more exercise. He wanted to go for a walk. I managed to settle him in front of the TV news while I got the children to bed, and then we went for a brief walk. It was raining hard, and we lived in a village with no pavements and no street lights, but we splashed through puddles for a couple of miles and then came home to a bath and bed ourselves. At midnight Clive was awake – he wanted to go for a walk. I persuaded him to stay put, and again twice more. When he woke me again at probably about 4 a.m. (it was still dark and still raining) and couldn't be dissuaded, I told him to get on with it and I would see him later, and went back to sleep. It was a mistake.

When I got up, about 8 a.m., there was no sign of Clive. The belt with the tracking device was still on the chair. At least it had stopped raining. I drove around, but there was no sign of him. I rang all the places he might have gone to (some of the day centres were in hospital grounds, and hence there was someone around on a Sunday morning). Finally, I rang the police, who were very sympathetic, and sent someone round very quickly to collect a photo of Clive and discuss a search strategy. They suggested sending up a helicopter to look for him, but I couldn't think of where to look, or what to look for. He had already been missing for several hours, and even in the dark that would mean he could be up to 20 miles away. Somehow I couldn't see Clive lying in a ditch with a broken leg.

The family next door came round to see what was going on, and, when they realised, were wonderfully helpful. He took all the children (theirs and mine) off to a local farm to see the lambs, and she made cups of tea, friendly small talk and lots of encouraging noises. The day dragged endlessly, but at last, just as it was getting dark, I got a phone call from the Swindon police. They hadn't heard Clive was missing (Thames Valley Police don't talk to other authorities, apparently), but they had found the address label Clive always carried, which had my phone number on. Clive had strayed onto the Swindon road, turned the wrong way, and just kept going, for about 30 miles. Some good neighbour in Swindon had seen how footsore he was, offered him a cup of tea, and called the police when they realised how poor his speech was. I intended to write to thank this good Samaritan, but never got round to it; if you're reading this, please accept both my thanks and my apologies. If you hadn't helped Clive then, he would have probably vanished into the crowd of homeless, and we would never have known what happened to him.

The police couldn't spare a car to bring Clive home, so I turned again to next door; they babysat the children while I drove to Swindon, found the police station, and saw Clive again. He was very pleased to see me, and hobbled out to the car for the drive home. I checked his feet that night; the soles were covered in blisters. He still got up the next day and went swimming!

The next day I backed my car into another while getting out of a crowded car park. It was obvious that we could no longer continue as we had done. I could just manage when Clive was independent for some of the day, but once he needed someone with him all the time, to stop him getting lost or wandering in front of a car, it was impossible. It would have been almost impossible if there had been just the two of us, but the children, then aged eight and nine, also needed me. Clive was due to go for respite in a fortnight; I got on the phone to the care home, and they agreed to take Clive permanently. I rang my boss and explained that I would not be in for the next two weeks, and concentrated on seeing that there were no disasters. I also had to label all Clive's clothes, and try to tell him that this time the respite would last a bit longer.

We managed to survive until the fateful day came. I didn't crash the car. No-one fell down stairs and broke their neck. The house didn't burn down, or get burgled. There were no floods or lightning strikes. I delivered Clive to the care home, and managed to drive home without hitting anything. Although the children were there to meet me, the house seemed very empty.

With hindsight

In the circumstances as they were, I think we did pretty well to keep going as long as we did, and with Clive as ill as he was. I continue to be amazed by his courage and ability to just keep going whatever the setbacks. Although at the time I felt very much on my own, it is clear that in fact I got a lot of help from neighbours, the people in OPTIMA, my GP, Clive's colleagues, and many others. What was not available was help for Clive, and this was because he did not want the sort of help that was then available. He didn't want anyone to help him get up, get dressed, get washed, or get about until the very late stages. What he needed was someone else who was familiar, knew Clive, knew about dementia, and could help him continue activities, and this someone needed to be able to get to know Clive, and needed

Clive to know and trust them, before the illness robbed him of the ability to learn new things and form new relationships. Such help was not then available. It is now through The Clive Project – more on this in Chapter 9.

We got through by taking each day as it came. Clive had his routine, so I only needed a few key words to remind him what to do. I tried to think what might go wrong, and how to avoid it. For example, everyone was worried about Clive's cycling. I made sure the bike was well-maintained, and had bike lights and reflectors. Clive always wore a helmet, and a reflective tape, and I stitched reflective strips into his clothes. He always had a note in his pocket with his address and telephone number on.

The Clive Project stemmed from the help provided for Clive by his colleagues, and organised for us by Steve, who remained (and still remains) in touch as Clive's illness progressed. Steve managed to cajole and persuade about a dozen of Clive's colleagues to give up the occasional Saturday to take Clive out. He organised a question-and answer session one evening, which Clive's consultant attended, where they could find out about Clive's illness and the difficulties it might cause. He organised a rota, and discussed the events of the day afterwards. Interestingly, they termed themselves a 'support group' and 'Friends of Clive', and that is exactly what they were. Someone would turn up in the middle of the morning and collect Clive. They took him out for a walk on the downs or by the river, or maybe for a pub lunch and a drive in the country, and delivered him back at tea-time. He obviously recognised his old friends and visibly enjoyed the outings. At the time I wasn't as anything like as grateful to his friends as I should have been; I'm sorry to say I was quite bad-tempered most of the time then, especially since I had to be calm and gentle in front of Clive and the children. I would like to thank everyone involved now – you know who you are, and your help was appreciated.

Many of the day centres Clive attended had to stretch their own rules to allow Clive to attend. I didn't realise the impact caring for Clive had on them until much later, and I'm very grateful that they were prepared to help. Clive was very much the same age as the volunteers and staff who ran the centres, whereas most of the other people who attended were a generation older. The manager at the Alzheimer's Club explained to me that, while they all felt very comfortable holding hands or exchanging a quick hug with someone elderly, it was different with someone the same age.

I wish help had been available to keep Clive at home with us for longer. At that stage he still knew us, and I think we could have managed a reasonable quality of life for all of us for another few months. But then, maybe I'm deluding myself. I was certainly close to breaking point.

Chapter 7

Nursing Homes

It's Christmas Day, and we have come to visit Clive in the nursing home, and bring him his presents. We opened our own presents at home, and had brunch – the home is over an hour's drive away but we had carols playing in the car, and it is a beautiful sunny winter's day. The home is near the downs, and snow is lying on the tops. We go in, and help Clive unwrap his presents – chocolates and a new dressing gown. The home is decorated for Christmas and looks very jolly, but there is only one sitting room, and everyone is there. Clive's bedroom is too small for all of us, so we go out for a walk. The sun is high, and the sky a very pale blue, but it is so cold. We stop in the swing park for a while, but even chasing each other around doesn't warm us up. We wander round the town, but the only places that are open won't admit children. It is Christmas Day, after all. We go back to the home and have a cup of hot chocolate, but I am so cold I feel as if I will never be warm again. The children are very subdued. One of the staff takes Clive off to change his wet shoes, and while he is distracted we get in the car and set off home. Merry Christmas to one and all.

Clive had stayed in the first care home twice before for respite; and was due to go for a third time when he started to get lost while out on his own. Although he knew the home, and they knew Clive, they imposed a new condition when they agreed to take him as a long-term resident: for the first six weeks they wanted no contact between Clive and any friends or family members. They explained that this was to help him settle in, and was their standard practice. I wasn't happy, and with hindsight I wish I hadn't agreed, but they were insistent. Their reasoning was that contact with home would make him feel very unsettled, but Clive was their first resident with dementia. Other people in the home were there to be taught how to live in society again while recovering from some trauma in their lives; Clive was there for a safe, secure and active environment, and, if he had been able to learn new skills, he wouldn't have needed to be there. But I didn't have a lot of choice. It was quite impossible for us to continue at home, and I had found no other place that would consider Clive, or that I would have considered for him. So we agreed. I left Clive at the home and set out on the 50-mile drive home. I did my best to explain to him, but he obviously didn't understand. He must have felt abandoned and betrayed by us all.

The six weeks went by very quickly for me. I was so tired and defeated by everything that just getting through the days was as much as I could manage. One of the OPTIMA nurses invited me round to supper; afterwards we had coffee and I joined them to help make a jigsaw. I had forgotten that such evenings were possible; it brought home to me how much my life had changed over the last two or three years. I was almost incapable of normal social interaction. I also took a week off entirely, and went diving in the Red Sea. The staff of the nursing home introduced me to the diving group. They knew I was a diver, as I had discussed them taking Clive diving on one of his respite visits. It was term-time, so I'm ashamed to say I farmed the children out to stay with school friends, and for a week I lived on a dive boat and did four or five dives every day, eating and reading in between dives, and sleeping under the stars. It was my first contact with diving and divers since I had broken my Achilles tendon, and it was solace for my soul. I had forgotten that such places existed, and that it was still possible for me to visit them. I took the children and my mother back to the Red Sea in October, but I still regret leaving them behind for that week. However, I needed the break.

Some time in the six weeks I got a telephone call from the staff at the home. What sedentary activity did Clive enjoy? I had to admit that he had never been one for sitting still if he could be moving about. He used to read a lot, and listen to the radio, and we played scrabble, but Clive was never one for jigsaws, or card games. They tried to get him interested in model-making, and I still have the kit for a model ship upstairs, but it has hardly been touched.

At the end of the six weeks, I went to visit Clive. At that stage, I still had dreams of Clive eventually being able to come home, so I wanted him to keep some contact with our house, and the village we lived in. I set out while the children were in school, collected Clive and brought him home. We collected the children from school together and spent the evening together; in the morning we took the children to school, Clive and I went for a walk together, and I took Clive back.

After a couple of weeks the people at the home were keen I should explain to Clive that he would be staying at the home for some time. So I arranged for someone (probably my mother, though I can't remember) to stay with the children, found what looked like a nice bed-and-breakfast not too far away from the home, and set out again. I collected Clive; we went for a walk on the downs, found the bed-and-breakfast, went for another walk to a pub for dinner, and had a pleasant, peaceful night together. It was mid-summer, and beautiful, warm, sunny weather. I tried to explain to Clive that I still loved him, and cared for him, but that looking after him at home was too much for me. I'm not sure he understood me; if he did I am sure he would not have agreed. Clive was such a self-reliant person that he never believed that he couldn't care for himself. So what if he got lost while out – did it really matter? Did we have the right to incarcerate him against his wishes for his own good? I wish I could have had that discussion with Clive before he was ill; as it was I just had to do the best that I could in the circumstances. Anyway, the next morning I took him back to the home; he walked in, and I drove home.

The home had refused to use the radio-tracking device. There was a lot of controversy then about using technology to replace staff in care homes, and I think they felt using the device would reflect badly on the home. They were also worried about the device upsetting Clive's pacemaker, and no-one could give them an absolute assurance that that wouldn't happen. They gave Clive a very active programme, including swimming every morning, and lots of walks, and trips to London. They even talked of trying to organise a diving session, though I don't think that ever proved possible. They certainly took him gliding, and to the seaside. I have photos of him beside the Cutty Sark, on the beach at Brighton, by the Thames Barrier. But Clive wanted to be at home, and he could be very determined. I got used to telephone calls to tell me 'Helen, we've lost Clive'. Normally he was found quite quickly, but on one occasion he managed to hitch a ride, and got 20 miles before he was found. Another time he was out practically all night. I got to see him as much as I could, but it was a hundred-mile round trip for every visit, and if I brought Clive home, it was two hundred miles. On one trip home the car broke down, and Clive was about to start marching off down the Oxford ring road when fortunately the engine started again. It was a very wet day, and I think the electrics had got a bit damp.

One morning the telephone rang on the dot of 6 a.m., and it was the home. Please could I talk to Clive? He was very distressed, and had been up all night, as he had decided I was going to divorce him. I tried to reassure him over the phone, and, as soon as the children were at school, I rang my boss to let him know I wouldn't be in, drove across to see Clive, and spent the day holding his hand and trying to show that I still loved him.

But, of course, eventually I had to leave him there, and go home to see to the children. I can't convey the despair and misery I felt as I left. I wanted to be with Clive, and look after him, show him I still loved him, and make the most of the time we had left. Yet I also wanted to be with the children, and they also needed me. I managed to drive home without hitting anything, which was something of a miracle. Clive's behaviour shows he was equally unhappy, and he could no longer understand why I was inflicting such misery on him.

The home was very small, and based in a normal family house. This was one of the reasons I had chosen it, as it was the sort of environment Clive was used to. It also meant that there was only one sitting room which the residents and staff shared, and so there was little privacy for family visits. I continued to bring Clive home for visits, and when it was the school holidays we all took Clive back. He didn't like being left, and so we had to wait until someone could distract Clive, or manage to take him out for a walk, and then we had to nip out and get away quickly. I often wondered what this type of visit – with the inability to say a proper farewell, and the deception involved – did to the children. It made me feel dreadful, and still does, but the only alternative was not visiting at all, which seemed much worse. I have asked them since, but they're not prepared to talk about anything connected with Clive's illness.

As Clive got worse, I stopped bringing him home, but instead went over for the day, and took him out for a walk and a pub lunch. We had many walks on the downs, watching the gliders from the local club. One day Clive was feeling amorous, so when we went back to the home I went upstairs to Clive's bedroom. Walking out again afterwards past the staff and other residents all tactfully looking the other way goes down as one of the most embarrassing moments of my life. He was my husband, and we had been married 25 years, yet I still felt like a cheap prostitute.

Our 25th wedding anniversary happened in the September of that year. I was puzzled what to do about it; I didn't want to pretend it was just another day, but Clive wasn't up to any major celebration. After much thought and consulting friends, I went across to see Clive on the anniversary itself, and took him out for a walk and a pub lunch. Then the children and I had a no-expenses-spared weekend in London. We checked into our hotel on Friday, and then went to see *Oliver*, where I had booked tickets in the front row of the stalls. The next morning the children discovered the delights of room service, and I had a peaceful delicious breakfast cooked by someone else. We fitted in as many of the London sights as possible, and on Saturday evening we went to see Jonathan Miller's *Mikado* at the English National Opera. Although not quite how I had imagined it 25 years ago, it was still a good anniversary.

All the time this was going on, I was also disputing with Social Services about paying for the nursing home. Although everyone (consultants, GP, Clive's social worker) had agreed that Clive had to be cared for elsewhere, and was too ill to remain at home, he was still expected to pay for his care out of his pension. I duly filled in the Social Services questionnaire, and some weeks later got their assessment. As Clive was no longer living at home, the Army had already cut his disability entitlement. I was entitled to half of Clive's basic pension; the children had no entitlement at all, but Social Services had allowed me a pittance for their care and proposed to take the rest (half of Clive's basic pension, and all the extras the Army had allowed because of his illness) to pay the nursing home fees. This seemed very unfair. Other places in the UK had hospital beds to care for people like Clive, but Oxfordshire had reorganised and closed them all. I had to fight the decision, or else be left with scarcely any money to raise the children. I can't remember who introduced me to Community Care Rights, a local charity funded by the Joseph Rowntree Foundation, who were my salvation. They showed me the Community Care Act, which had come into being to cover cases like Clive's, yet Clive's social worker had never heard of it. They helped me to collect the evidence needed to show that Clive's care should be funded by the NHS; they represented me at the much-delayed hearing which finally met to consider Clive's case, and won for me an agreement that the costs of Clive's care would be met by the NHS. Fighting this battle took an extraordinary amount of my time and energies, and lasted from March, when Clive went into care, until the middle of August. Although that meant that the bills would be paid in the future, Social Services still tried to get me to pay for Clive's care up till then; it took another six months before they finally agreed that there had been undue delay on their part, and they would not expect me to pay the bills. I had already paid the total amount for the first two weeks, as that had been arranged by me before Social Services became involved. I have since been told that I should have been able to claim some help with all the travelling expenses I had to pay, but I never managed to find a way.

There is a strange dichotomy in England in that hospital treatment is absolutely free to the person receiving it, and if someone with dementia can no longer be cared for at home and is instead receiving care in the local hospital they do not have to pay. However, if the local hospital has closed the beds that used to be available, so that care is given in a nursing home, that care has to be paid for. Since a young person with dementia often needs a lot of care, this can be very expensive. When the system was first introduced, if the person in care had a pension, the nursing home was entitled to claim all of the pension to pay the fees. After a lot of complaints about the unfairness of this, a new rule was brought in that allowed the partner of the person in care half of the pension to meet their own needs. Probably because few people in this position had dependent children, no such entitlement was made for children. This is still the case.

Although things have improved since Clive first went into care, I still meet many people at conferences and through The Clive Project who have the same worries and heartbreak that I had. It is very painful to admit that the partner you planned to spend your life with needs more care than you can provide, and having to pay for the care you wish you did not need rubs salt in the wound.

It was a very cold winter that year; there was snow before Christmas and it stayed icy and treacherous underfoot well into January. To make matters worse, as well as staff absences over the holiday season, there was a flu epidemic, which made the home even shorter of staff. There were not enough people to take Clive out, and in any event it was actually quite dangerous to walk anywhere, as things were so slippery. However, one could not explain any of these things to Clive, who wanted to go for a walk. As I've already said, the home was in a normal family house, with an obvious front door and back door. Clive wanted to go out; there was no-one to take him, and it was not safe for him to go on his own. He could not be distracted, so the doors were locked. It was never a good plan to try and stop Clive physically from doing something he wanted to do, and he reacted predictably: he picked up a fire extinguisher and broke out.

Understandable and predictable as Clive's reaction was, it was also entirely unacceptable, and the staff at the home reacted in another predictable and understandable way: Clive was prescribed fairly substantial doses of a sedative to calm him down and make him easier to manage.

Before this happened, I had already begun to look for another home for Clive. The first home had been the best that was available for Clive at the time, but his illness had continued to worsen, and his abilities to understand what was going on around him, and react accordingly, were noticeably less than they had been nine months before. He was the first resident suffering from dementia that the home had cared for, and I felt they didn't really understand how to care for him. It was also a long way for me to drive, and there was no privacy for the family on visits. The ever-helpful OPTIMA people suggested I visit a home near Banbury.

This was a home set in a large house in a small village. It catered especially for people with dementia, and, although most of the residents were much older than Clive, the owner and staff were sure they would be able to cope. They had to apply for special permission to take Clive as a resident, as he was under 65 (in fact, he was 49 by now). They also had a policy which appealed to me, of no inappropriate use of drugs. I took Clive on a visit, and again I have no idea how much he understood of what was going on, but it seemed worthwhile to try out a move. The new home gave him a huge room with an attached bathroom, in an annex attached to the main house. They even looked out an exercise bike, in case Clive could remember how to cycle.

I took along photos and mementos from home to make the place seem as familiar as possible. Social Services agreed to fund the new home, and even to fund both places for two weeks, in case Clive would not settle at the new place. I transferred him in February. It was still a cold, hard winter, but spring was not far away. The new home worked out well from the start for me, and I think Clive was happier as well. It was much easier to visit; the drive was normally less than half an hour, instead of nearly an hour, and the driving was much easier. We could visit Clive without seeing anyone else except staff, and there was plenty of space in his room for us all to sit. In bad weather, there were several walking circuits in the main house, where Clive could walk all day without upsetting anyone, and the house was surrounded by big gardens, and then mostly by open fields. It was close to the main road through the village, which could be extremely busy at rush hour, but there was a long drive and a barrier to deter people from wandering out that way. The staff at this home were also prepared to use the tracking device, so the Oxford academic whose pet project it was went along with the belt and aerial, to show the staff how it worked.

I used to visit Clive once a week on my own, and if the weather was reasonable we went for a walk. We often went to the Oxford canal, where I was certain I wouldn't get lost. When we first started going, the narrowboats that were moored there were iced-in, and the ones used as permanent residences often had wood-burning stoves going, sending up the lovely scent of woodsmoke. Gradually the ice thawed, the towpath got less treacherous, and we could walk further. The trees and bushes greened, and then the swallows and swifts arrived. I loved to see them flying along the canal, dipping into the water to take a drink, and wheeling to and fro in a wonderful display of con- trolled flying, as they hunted insects. Mud banks became covered in primroses and coltsfoot, and then daisies and bugle. The nettles and brambles in the hedges began to grow across the towpath, so we often had to walk in single file. I don't know about Clive, but I found some sort of peace in these walks together; I think he did too. There were times when he marched ahead, but mostly he walked nearby, and, on occasion, where there was room to walk side by side I was allowed to hold his hand. He was certainly always happy to come out with me. As summer progressed, we often stopped and bought an ice-cream in the post office of the village where I parked, which had a convenient bench outside where we could rest our sore feet. One memorable day we walked into Banbury and back. There is an enormous bridge where the M40 crosses the canal, giving an interesting contrast of old and new technology.

Most weekends I visited with the children. Sometimes we also went to the canal, or walked about the village, or just mooched about in Clive's room or the gardens of the home. There were often other residents about in the garden, and their behaviour could be bizarre, yet the children did not seem upset or worried in any way. On one occasion I forgot to lock the car, and when we returned we found it full of old dears who were waiting eagerly to be taken on an outing.

Clive still went wandering, either along the drive and past the barrier, or over the six-foot-high stone wall that surrounded the garden. Mostly Clive wore the belt, and the staff located him quite quickly. As long as he was safe, they let him walk for an hour or so, and then drove alongside and 'accidentally' noticed him and offered him a lift home. He was tired by then, and happy to go back.

Alas, one time in the Easter holidays he went out without the belt, and could not be found. When it got dark, the home rang me to let me know, and I waited on tenterhooks by the phone. We were due to go on holiday the next day, to visit relatives in the States. The tickets were booked and the bags packed; we were expecting to leave early the next morning. I was travelling with my mother and the children. I thought through the possibilities. Rachel was 9, Alan 8 and my mother 77. Although they were all confident and capable, I just could not see them getting to the airport, crossing the Atlantic and managing the luggage without me. The relatives we were visiting were my mother's age, and one was already showing early signs of Alzheimer's disease. I reluctantly decided that if I couldn't go neither could the children. Our tickets were non-transferrable, so if we didn't go the next day we didn't go at all. Our travel insurance would not cover a cancellation due to a pre-existing condition. The telephone rang just before 11 p.m. Clive had wandered miles from the home, and strayed onto the busy dual carriageway between Banbury and Northampton. He was walking along the side of the road, but almost invisible in the dark, and had been hit by a lorry. Fortunately the lorry had just caught Clive with the wing mirror, and the driver had stopped immediately, found Clive on the side of the road and called the police. Clive was at Banbury Hospital with a broken arm. Once again, I felt torn in two. I really wanted to go and see Clive, to reassure myself he was alright, and to hold his hand. The matron of the home was at the hospital, and she urged me strongly not to come. Clive was sedated and asleep for the night, she told me. He was fine apart from the broken arm (his right arm, as luck would have it – he was right-handed). It was a clean break, and he would be discharged and back at the home the next day. I allowed myself to be persuaded, and set off the next day to the States.

We had a good holiday. We saw many of the tourist sights in Washington – the White House, the Treasury, the Vietnam Memorial and the Space Museum – yet the bit that most sticks in my mind is taking Alan and Rachel out to the Shenandoah Valley. Clive and I had spent a magic few days there 20 years earlier, and the magic was still there. Alas, the balmy autumn weather that Clive and I had enjoyed was not there. The day before we had been sitting on the patio in T-shirts; the day we spent in Shenandoah it snowed and the wind was bitterly cold. I don't think it is my children's favourite place, but I will take them back some time when the weather is likely to be better.

Back in England, we went to see Clive as soon as possible. He looked well apart from the cast on his arm. It had already been replaced twice, as he didn't like it and had managed to destroy two plaster casts in the ten days we had been away. Although things seemed OK, over the next few days I realised he was no longer the happy-go-lucky person he had managed to remain. We had to go to Oxford to get Clive's glasses checked, and, when he was hemmed in by a crowd of people, he used the cast on his arm as a flail to clear a way. Fortunately no-one was hurt, but I was very alarmed. I wished more than ever that I had been able to visit him in hospital just after his accident, but that might have made no difference. Even so, I couldn't blame Clive if he thought that I had abandoned him.

Not very long afterwards, I got home to find a message on the answerphone asking me to ring the home. The matron explained that she had felt that they could no longer care for Clive properly, and so, after discussion with Clive's consultant, he had been sectioned under the Mental Health Act, and then moved to the local hospital, where a new centre had just opened to care for people with Alzheimer's disease. The point of the sectioning was that it gave the consultant the right to move him, and also emphasised that, in their opinion, Clive was incapable of making decisions about his own care.

The new centre was a beautiful place, built behind the main hospital, and totally separate; it even had a separate driveway and car park. It was built in a square round a sunny courtyard, with single rooms for all the residents, a kitchen where visitors could make tea and coffee, and lots of alcoves for people to sit. It took about 15 people at once, and had a lot of staff. It ought to have felt OK, but it didn't, probably because of the circumstances under which Clive was admitted. They initially sedated him quite heavily, and when they lessened the medication Clive had lost the little language he had retained, and showed no signs of knowing who I was, or of recognising his own children. Although I knew this might happen, nothing had prepared me for the grief I would feel. It was another loss on top of so many at that time. But Clive would still sit and tolerate my holding his hand, so I spent a long time sitting in the sun with him, trying to make the most of the new situation.

As I said, the new unit was built around a square, and Clive walked for hours round and round the square. Unfortunately one of the other residents took exception to this, and tried to stop Clive by standing in front of him. Apparently (I wasn't there at the time), Clive gave him one push to get him out of the way, and then continued his walk. The other man lost his balance, fell over and fractured his hip. He recovered, but it made everyone very wary of Clive. Despite that, a few days later when Clive's mother and stepfather came to visit they were encouraged to try and move Clive out of one of the alcoves, where he was sitting in the sun, and into his own room where there would be more privacy. Clive no longer understood any spoken requests, so his stepfather tried to pull Clive to his feet, and again got pushed over. He also broke his hip, though he managed to drive another hundred miles before finding out. So things were fairly disastrous there. I suppose Clive spent a couple of months there, and then he was moved again, to a similar unit in Oxford where a place had just become free. And so Clive came to his final home.

With hindsight

Clive went into the first nursing home in April 1997, nearly ten years ago as I write this. In some ways things have changed for the better; in other ways they have got worse. There are now a few homes scattered around the country which cater specifically for people with younger onset dementia. There are not many of them, and they all have waiting lists as long as they are prepared to take, but they do exist. Most of them do not do respite care, but again there are a few specialised units which do. The homes which care for the elderly patients with dementia are often closing down, faced with increasing regulation and under-funding.

The question of funding a place in a specialist care facility is yet another problem. It seems inconceivable nowadays that there should be no national standards that define who is eligible for NHS care and who is not. I have talked to very few people who have managed to get NHS continuing care funding for their partner without a long and protracted battle, and even fewer who manage to get care to keep someone with dementia in their own home for as long as possible. Clive could maybe have had another six months of living at home with his family, if care could have been arranged. It just seems so unfair that the family who are already facing losing one family member should also face a hard financial battle, or else live in penury in order to pay the nursing home fees. There is a real postcode lottery, and no-one apart from the families involved and a few organisations such as the Alzheimer's Society seem to care. I know people who have moved house in order to get to an area with better care provision. If nursing home fees have to be paid by the family of the person with dementia, there is no provision made within the law to set aside a proportion of the family income to provide for children. A spouse is entitled to a certain proportion of any pension, but children are not entitled to a penny. This seems very unfair.

One of the biggest points of discussion was the risks we allowed Clive to take. This was always an issue, but when he was living at home I could control things more easily. Many people criticised me for allowing Clive as much freedom as I did, but I had a very clear view that Clive should not be stopped from doing things unless he was endangering others directly. A small part of the reason was that stopping Clive from doing anything he wanted to do was very difficult, but mostly it was a recognition that before he was ill he was a risk taker. His hobbies were always active, and potentially dangerous – skydiving, skiing, fell-walking, scuba diving, running marathons. He was an active, energetic person, and that didn't suddenly change when he became ill.

While driving to and from the various homes, I used to dream about the best place for Clive, assuming it wasn't feasible for him to live at home. Discussions with others in The Clive Project crystallised these ideas, so, with thanks to those others, here is my recipe for the ideal nursing home designed to care for people with dementia, whatever their age. While there is nothing here that is specific to younger people rather than older people, the experience of the second home Clive stayed in made it clear that younger people with dementia do not always mix happily with the frail elderly.

The ideal home would offer a base to all people with dementia, whatever the stage of their illness. Hence it could be used for a day centre and occasional respite breaks for those in the early stages, more supportive accommodation for those in need of it, and hospice and palliative care for those in the end stages. The staff should know about dementia, but recognise that people with dementia can still have a good quality of life. The rooms would be organised in smallish clusters, preferably around a sitting area with space and equipment for tea- and coffee-making. Clusters should be easily distinguished one from another – maybe by differing decoration – yet things like light switches should be in the same position throughout. There should be space for at least one uninterrupted walking circuit – one inside and one outside would be ideal. There should be an enclosed, safe garden where people could sit in the sun, or help with the gardening if they wanted (not Clive ever!). Bedrooms should all be en-suite, and big enough for a visitor or two to sit in comfort. The place should be close enough to other facilities for access by walking – for example, swimming pool, sports centre, shops and cafes, cinema. There should be easy access for visitors, yet the place should be reasonably secure against intruders. The place should have a friendly, welcoming, non-institutional feel. The staff should be prepared to work in partnership with other organisations (e.g. The Clive Project) who could offer extra activities. People with dementia should be encouraged to do what they can, and reassured that they will not be judged. Their input, and that of their families, should be sought.

And if all this seems like hoping for flying pigs, I do know of nursing homes that offer it. If they can do it, why can't every home?

Chapter 8

Final
Harbour

Clive is half-sitting, half-lying on the sofa when I walk in. He is alone in the room – a small sitting room with The Beatles playing on the stereo. Most of the others are in the big sitting room, listening to Bing Crosby. I pull up a chair and sit next to him. He no longer recognises me, but sometimes he lets me hold his hand. Today is one of those days. I tell him what the children and I are up to. I don't think he understands any of it, but you can never tell. It seems more comfortable to me than just sitting in silence, though I do sit quietly for a while as well. When he starts to get restless, I get his shoes on, and we go out for a walk round the hospital. In the past we have walked all the way round the hospital, which is probably about a mile, but today we just wander across to the golf course. I used to take Clive across the bridge and through a field full of wild flowers, but there is a stile on the way, and I no longer dare try to get him across. He has lost the coordination needed to climb a stile. The sun is warm on our backs. We wander for a few minutes, then go back to the centre. The staff welcome Clive with a cup of tea. I give him a hug and say goodbye – I need to go to collect the children from school. I don't know if Clive gets anything from these visits, but I feel a compulsion to visit as often as I can – not every day, but several times every week. I like to think he appreciates the visits as well, and has just lost the ability to express that.

The Oxford centre was again a new unit, built behind one of the big hospitals in Headington. It had three wards within the main building; Clive was given a place in the most secure unit, where the doors were kept locked. Clive was moved there by ambulance, so I didn't have to drive him, but I was there to meet him and try to help get him settled. Again, he had his own room, light and airy, with plenty of space for his bed and a couple of armchairs. This ward was also built round a courtyard, but the courtyard was filled with a very pleasant garden and a small fountain, and there was a doorway out. The water in the fountain was sometimes dyed to give a bit of variety; blue and green looked good, but red was rather ghoulish, though it very much entertained the children. I liked it from the beginning; it had a very friendly feel to it.

The unit was supposedly a short-stay ward. It had been built specifically to look after people with dementia. The idea had been to take people who were not settling in a nursing home, or proving difficult to care for, to find the reasons for the behaviour, to sort out any *necessary* medication (they did not have a policy of heavy sedation), and then move them on somewhere else. It was a good idea; the only problem was that there were very few other suitable homes. Many of their residents stayed for months or years. For the first two or three months that Clive was there, the ward manager kept arranging meetings to discuss 'Clive's onward placement'. I wasn't particularly worried by any of these meetings. At each one, I explained that I had no ideas of any home anywhere that would consider taking Clive as a resident. If they could suggest anywhere, I would happily go and look. They never did come up with any suggestions, and eventually accepted that Clive was there to stay, and stopped calling meetings.

It's difficult to say why this ward felt so much friendlier than any of the other places Clive stayed. There was a similar feel to the second home, but that was very much bigger than this ward. It was as if everyone connected to the ward belonged to one very large extended family, which had some very eccentric members, and everyone was accepted and appreciated.

The difference in attitude was brought home to me when, in the first few days he was there, Clive managed to get out. I didn't get a frantic phone call to tell me they had lost him. Instead, when I came along later that afternoon, Clive was sitting in a chair with his feet up with a cup of tea and a biscuit. Tea was quickly made for me, and then Clive's allocated nurse told me the tale. They had missed Clive shortly after lunch. They presumed he had managed to climb out of a small open window, and had been gone about half an hour. Search parties were organised, and one of them found Clive walking down the main street of Headington, nearly two miles away, in his stockinged feet. The overall feeling was one of understanding that he did not like being caged, and admiration that he had managed to evade them, and get so far in such a short time. Later there was an enquiry into how he had managed to get out, and things were changed to try and avoid a repeat, but no-one was angry with Clive, and no-one expressed any frustration or annoyance to him or to me. Although by this time Clive had no language left at all, he could still sing, and continued to sing snatches of the three songs that had set the theme for the last few years. He had always loved Edith Piaf's *Non, je ne regrette rien*, although Clive's rendition was not one you would pay money to hear. Another favourite was Engelbert Humperdinck's *Please Release Me*, and the third was Roy Orbison's *Only the Lonely*. I often wondered if it was sheer chance that these songs stuck in his mind, or if he was trying to tell us something. It is well known that people who have lost one language can retain another, and that the ability to sing stays for a long time. However, another song was added to Clive's repertory in this ward: he could often be seen walking round the circuit with the ward sister, both singing *Daisy, Daisy*. She was a lovely Irish lady, who set the tone for the whole ward in a wonderfully friendly, inclusive way. All the staff made a point of getting to know Clive's family, and seemed genuinely interested in us, as well as trying to understand Clive through us.

As I said, the ward was designed around a courtyard, and the main corridor ran right round the building. However, unlike the previous unit, the corridor had been designed to be unobtrusive. The seating in the sitting rooms faced out to the gardens surrounding the ward, so Clive could and did walk for hours without disturbing anyone. The only badly designed feature was the fire doors. Fire doors in many hospitals are normally open, and close automatically if the fire alarm goes off. These were designed to be closed, and had to be opened manually to get through them. This wasn't a problem at first, but as Clive deteriorated still further he couldn't work out how to open the door, and would stand next to it for a long time, trying various strategies. He never gave up; if no-one opened the door for him he would persevere until he succeeded.

They realised very quickly that Clive loved to be out in the fresh air, and tried to take him for a walk every morning. If the weather was bad, or they were short-staffed, they would get him to settle in the courtyard garden. If he spent some time outside every morning, he would then mostly settle in a chair for at least a few hours in the afternoon. His illness meant that he slept a lot more than normal, and he was also by now prepared to watch TV. Clive normally sat in a smaller sitting room, with only one or two of the other residents. The ward did not have a policy of constant music, but, if music was played, in the bigger sitting room it was music for my parent's generation – Bing Crosby, Vera Lynn, and their ilk. In the small sitting room, it was always the music that had been popular in Clive's youth – The Beatles, The Rolling

Stones, and so on. We brought tapes in for them to play, but the staff also provided some of their own.

For his birthday present, I found a machine that could display disco-style light effects, which we set up in his bedroom. I'm told he enjoyed watching the colours moving about the walls and ceiling; certainly the children and I did. The walls of his room were decorated with photos of his family, and pictures drawn and painted by the children.

Some time after Clive had been sectioned, there was a big meeting to discuss renewing the section. I can't remember if it was six months or a year after the original admission, and the law governing that has probably changed since then. It was a serious meeting, with me, a solicitor representing Clive, Clive's consultant and the unit matron, and the pros and cons of the renewal were discussed in great depth. I was impressed, and reassured. This was, after all, giving the staff the right to hold and treat Clive against his will. As it happened, in Clive's case there was no conflict. Clive couldn't express his wishes, but everyone including me was sure he was unsafe outside the unit, and there was no question of undue sedation or any potentially harmful treatment. I still found it very comforting that such a big decision was not taken lightly by anyone.

And so we settled into another routine. There were no official visiting hours, and there was a convenient car park just outside, so I got into the habit of dropping by nearly every day, often only for a few minutes. I would sit with Clive, and hold his hand if he would let me, and we would look at photographs, or I would tell him what was happening in our lives. Sometimes we just sat together. Once or twice a week I would go for a longer visit, and take Clive out for a walk. There was a golf course next to the hospital, and quite a lot of open ground, and to begin with we often made a circuit of the hospital. As time went by, our walks got slower and we covered less ground. One of our regular walks led over a stile and a footbridge over a stream, and once I was worried I would not be able to get Clive back, as he seemed disturbed by the water flowing underneath the footbridge, and couldn't work out how to get across the stile. I had visions of having to leave Clive to go and get help, and coming back to find him gone. But he managed in the end.

I allowed the children to dictate when and if they wanted to visit. If they wanted to go, I would always try and take them as soon as possible, and the staff always made them very welcome, and let them join in any activity that was arranged. There was often a baking session going on, with delectable smells coming from the kitchen. However, these visits became less and less frequent. I could understand why: Clive did not recognise them, and I remember hating visiting my own parents when they were ill, even though they knew me and could talk to me. Sometimes I dropped in on our way back from somewhere else, if I was nearby. On these occasions, the children often chose to stay in the car, or come inside and sit in the unit's reception area.

The food in the ward was deliberately very plain and English, as that was what most of the residents were used to. Clive preferred his food very spicy and so they tried to allow for this. Someone would go out for a Chinese or Indian take-away, and they allowed me to fill one drawer of the freezer with very garlicky curry or lasagne. And I took in a cafetière and ground coffee, so Clive could have the very strong black coffee he preferred. He only drank coffee at breakfast or lunchtime, avoiding it in the evenings as it kept him awake. I often saw him dozing off at lunchtime with the coffee cup still in his hand, so I never quite believed this, but I never contradicted him.

Clive continued slowly to deteriorate. He sang more rarely. He walked much more slowly, and started tripping over things. He needed more help dressing and feeding himself. He allowed someone to shave him by now, so he was once again the smooth-faced Clive I remembered, but there was no spark of recognition in his eyes when I went to see him. The arm he had broken started hurting him – he couldn't tell us, but you could see from the way he held it, and the fingers of that hand started turning inwards, like someone playing a violin. He still walked round and round the circuit, but he had great difficulty with the fire doors, and eventually started walking into them with a great 'thud', but he shook his head, recovered and continued walking, keeping going in the same direction if someone opened the door, or turning around otherwise. Changing direction was obviously difficult – he would shuffle around in a confused manner for a few seconds before he set off again. It seemed to be some inner compulsion that kept him moving. He lost a lot of weight, despite all attempts to tempt him with food he liked, until he was just skin and bone. He had difficulty swallowing, and often choked on his food.

At the ward's request, I got some velcro slippers for him. Clive had never liked slippers; indoors he always used to wear socks, or just wander around barefoot. I did not expect the slippers to be successful, but it was worth a try. We hoped he would trip less often with them on, and they would protect his feet. Alas, Clive could always work out a way to remove them. He was less prepared now to let me hold his hand; if I picked it up he would pull away.

Winter came and went. We could very rarely get far on our walks now, but I still tried to get Clive outside for a few minutes. One spring day, with the sun shining, I decided to take him up to a local beauty spot to see the apple blossom. It was really difficult to get Clive into the car, as he had forgotten how. One of the nurses tickled his tummy to try and persuade him to bend in the middle. We managed to get him in safely, and I drove up to the top of the hill to admire the view and enjoy the sunshine. I didn't dare to try and get Clive out for a walk, though that had been my original intention. We stayed there in peace for an hour or so, then went back to the ward for tea.

A few weeks later, I was sitting in the office when I got a phone call from the ward. Clive was not well, and please could I come over. I made apologies to my boss, and set out. I remember on the way there I missed the road, and ended up in a housing estate behind the dust cart. The road was not wide enough for me to overtake, and I felt if I tried to do a three-point turn I might hit something, so I just waited fatalistically until it was out of the way. When I finally reached the ward, I could see at a glance that Clive was not well. He was very flushed, and coughing. The nurses thought he had pneumonia, and wanted to know what they should do. If I wanted them to try and treat the illness, Clive would have to be transferred to the main hospital, and treated with intravenous antibiotics. If he recovered, he would then face a long convalescence. Alternatively, he could stay in the ward, and they would provide palliative care, but not attempt to treat the infection.

This wasn't a decision I felt prepared to make on my own. I knew what my feelings were, but I had to consult Clive's family. The ward made an office and telephone available, and I started making telephone calls. Clive's mother, brother and sister all came across in the next day or two, and we were unanimous in deciding to keep Clive where he was. He was as familiar with the place and the people as he was capable of; they knew and under-stood him, and his quality of life seemed pretty poor before he was ill. Later that day he was being hoisted out of bed to be bathed and have the sheets changed, and he tried desperately to stand to attention. It was almost his last conscious act.

Fortunately the ward was very close to a hospice, so when Clive seemed to be in some pain later, the hospice could provide a morphine pump to keep him comfortable. The staff did their best to keep him comfortable, and to care for his family. One of the nurses took the children for breakfast at McDonald's while I stayed with Clive. They found beds for his mother and me to stay. They certainly gave Clive all the care and love they had. On the last day, I took the children to see him, and then took them home where a neighbour stayed with them. Clive slipped slowly away at 2 a.m. on 29 April 1999.

I couldn't believe it, and I still find it difficult. Clive had always been so alive, so determined to keep himself fit, so strong, so healthy. Even when he fell ill, the illness affected his mind and not his body until the very late stages. Even when the ward called me in, and I could see how ill he was, I expected him to fight off this illness as he had fought and won so many battles in the previous few years. Even as I was sitting there in the last few hours listening to the inconstant, struggling breaths, I never really believed he would leave me. I sat in the room with the silent, emaciated thing that had been Clive, and held his cold hand for one last time. Then I gave his mother a hug, and went home to our children.

Of course I kept going. I owed it to Clive and the children and myself. The hospital arranged for a post-mortem as part of the research Clive had been involved in. His mother had not been keen on the idea, but the rest of the family were united that this was what Clive had wanted, and that it was important to the rest of us to know as much as possible about his illness.

Clive was buried in the local churchyard. It was a promise I had made to myself when he had to go into a nursing home, and kept trying to get home, that at the end I would get him as close to home as I could. There was a good turnout for his funeral. His Army colleagues did him proud, and one of the nurses from the ward talked about the 'generous, funny Clive' that they had known. I wished they could have known him in his prime. I didn't realise it, but one of the hymns I had chosen had two possible tunes. After a few initial chords, the organist launched into one, and the congregation into the other. We battled it out for the first verse, and then the rector stopped the fight, and declared that we would sing the whole hymn unaccompanied. I could just picture Clive hooting with laughter at the spectacle. We did our best to lift the roof off the small village church.

I was used to going into a house without Clive – he had been in care for the last three years. But going home still felt very different, and very lonely. I now had to face was the prospect of a life without Clive. He had been my rock, my friend, my lover, the father of my children, and now he was gone. It was the nature of

Army life that we moved frequently, and while I had made some very good friends, few of them lived nearby. When the children were born, and I would naturally have expected to make more friends, Clive was beginning to be ill. He had been the focus of my life for nearly 30 years, and without him I was nothing.

I slowly reinvented my life, saved mostly by the children. However little I felt like getting up in the morning, they gave me a reason. If I just wanted to sit at home and cry, they didn't allow me to. However, there was one subject I wasn't allowed to talk about. I used to talk about Clive, to tell them how much he had loved them as babies, and how he would have taken them on holidays, or to school outings. Finally my daughter, then aged 11, turned to me. 'Look Mum', she said forcefully, 'I don't want to hear about the wonderful dad I haven't got'. So I shut up. I hope they will be more interested in him later on, when they feel ready. And if that's never, well that's their choice.

There was little paperwork to do following Clive's death – only registering the death and sorting out the insurance policies. All the important things had been done when we realised he was ill. In many ways, some people would say that Clive died back then, in his ability to function as a responsible adult in society. The next six years allowed the body to catch up with the mind. And yet Clive was in no way dead while he was ill. He still had a sense of humour; until the last year or so he enjoyed the company of his family; he liked to go out to the theatre, to theme parks, for a walk in the country, to feed the ducks with his family. He was immensely proud of his children; he liked to be with his colleagues; he liked to go to the pub even though he gave up alcohol as soon as he was diagnosed. He loved to go swimming. He loved life. And I think he fitted as much into his 51 years as was possible.

With hindsight

The post-mortem showed that Clive's final illness was not pneumonia, but endocarditis – an infection of the heart valves probably caused by his pacemaker in combination with the extreme weight loss he suffered in the last few months. This is an even more serious illness, and makes me doubly glad that we decided not to try and treat it. The underlying dementia was diagnosed as cortico-basal dementia. This is extremely rare; there is no known cause, and still no understanding of the illness and no prospect of a cure. Fortunately, there is also no suggestion that it is inheritable.

The ward where Clive spent his final months has been expanded. The wonderful ward sister has retired and gone home to Ireland, and most of the rest of the staff who cared for Clive have moved on. It now copes with almost twice as many patients with the same number of staff. They no longer have the space they had; I don't know if they still have a kitchen where residents and families can make tea and cook biscuits. I am no longer in touch, but I hope that the staff have managed to develop the sense of being a family that made their care of Clive so exceptional, and helped us all come to terms with what was happening to him.

Chapter 9

Start of The Clive Project

It's an evening in October 1999, six months after Clive died. I'm in the palatial surroundings of a function room at Headington Hall. It has tremendously high ceilings, ornate plaster coving and ceiling roses and heavy chintz curtains. Earlier there was a tremendous view across the surrounding park to Oxford, but it's getting dark and we've drawn the curtains. Strange to think that not very long ago this was a family house; now it is part of Oxford Brookes University and they have kindly allowed us to use the room. There are about 40 of us – members of The Clive Project steering group, support workers, people with dementia and their families. The Clive Project has been providing one-to-one support for a year now, and we're celebrating. It is not a wild party. We share the food we have brought, and chat about this and that. A musician friend has volunteered some of his friends to come and play for us. After supper we try and have a more serious discussion about how The Clive Project should develop. Most people are happy with the support they receive, but want more hours. Somebody wants The Project's next birthday party to be in the Caribbean! Somebody else produces a magnificent birthday cake, and we raise our glasses in celebration. It's time to go, but no-one seems to want to leave. We slowly move from the chairs to cluster around the door to the room, then around the cloakroom outside, then in the car park. Everyone is too busy chatting to want to go home.

The Clive Project started quietly, as a research project funded by the Oxfordshire branch of the Alzheimer's Society. Some of their members had been struck by the lack of appropriate support for Clive and other younger people with dementia within Oxfordshire, and decided to do something. They invited me to join them, and I agreed. When the meetings first started, they were held at lunchtime on one of the days Clive was at a day centre. Later he was in a nursing home, but we still met at lunchtime, when the children were at school.

Younger onset dementia was beginning to get a slightly higher profile than in the past; there were some research papers, including a very good one by Richard Harvey on the prevalence of the illness.[1] However, our group included someone from the local Social Services, and she told us quite forcefully that we would never be able to persuade anyone to provide any services unless we could point out the people who needed them. So the first step was to hire a part-time researcher to identify the people with young-onset dementia. It wasn't as easy a job as it sounds, and is symptomatic of the difficulties of providing care for this group. Clive was diagnosed by a neurologist, but others were diagnosed by psychiatrists or by geriatricians. And as there were no services and no treatment, once the diagnosis had been made general care was often provided by GPs, as with Clive, and there are a lot of GPs within Oxfordshire, and they don't all have

[1]   Harvey, R., Skelton-Robinson, M., and Rossor, M.N. (2003) 'The prevalence and causes of dementia in people under the age of 65 years.' *Journal of Neurologyy, Neurosurgery, and Psychiatry 74*, 1206–1209. Available at http://jnnp.bmj.com/cgi/content/full/74/9/1206, accessed on 28 August 2008.

time to talk to researchers. In fact, in her first trawl through the likely sources of names, our researcher missed one Clive Beaumont, despite her having talked to the supervisor of Clive's social worker. However, with a lot of perseverance, she eventually came up with a list of over 30 names, which seemed to us sufficient to prove the need for some sort of service.

We spent the next few meetings talking about the sort of service that might help. We discussed information websites, and decided they were difficult to maintain, and in any event likely to be used by the family and friends of the person with dementia, and we really wanted to focus on helping the person with dementia. We considered a day centre providing more active care then the day centres for the elderly, but, with a small, geographically spread group, it was difficult to think of a convenient place without everyone spending hours travelling. Then I remembered how Clive's colleagues had come to take him out, and suggested we try to provide this sort of care. Everyone agreed it was a good idea, and we spent the next few meetings discussing how such an idea might work. Our researcher discussed the possibility with other people with dementia, and their families and friends. The idea was favourably received. 'Good idea' they said. 'When do you start?'

We agreed very early on that the care would only work if it was consistent (same service provider, regular appointments, good timekeeping) and tailored to the needs of the person with dementia, and that the service provider needed some training in what living with dementia meant to the person and their family and friends. We agreed that three hours seemed a reasonable length for a session – longer and we were likely to exhaust the person with dementia; shorter and we were not going to achieve very much for anyone.

We devised a training programme for potential service providers, and then sat back and looked at our Social Services rep. After all, we felt, we had done all her work for her. She had a list of names of people in need of these services; she had a model of the service – all she had to do was start things off.

'Good idea' she said. 'We'd really like to do this, *but* we haven't any money. Maybe next year.'

Well, that didn't sound good to us. We were trying to provide help for people with a progressive illness. Clive was already in a home, and beyond such help. If we waited a year, how many other names would have dropped off the list, and would we then have to wait another six months while our intrepid researcher identified the next lot? After all, while these illnesses are rare, they are unfortunately not that rare. In fact, Richard Harvey's figures suggested there might be about 200 people with younger onset dementia living within Oxfordshire.

We asked our researcher to change tack. Instead of writing letters to hospital consultants and social workers, we asked her to write to charitable organisations. It immediately became clear that we had to break with the Alzheimer's Society; they couldn't fund us directly themselves, but, while we were attached to them, we had difficulty fund-raising on our own. And then one of the local charitable funds offered to give us enough money to start a service!

We sat at the next meeting looking rather thunderstruck. This was a big step we were considering. We wouldn't be a local research and campaigning group any more. Were we really prepared to take the responsibility of employing support workers, with all that involved in the way of tax and insurance, and then to provide an adequate service for people with dementia and their families? I was quite adamant that we should not go ahead unless we were confident the whole thing would work, at least for a while. I had been disappointed too many times to wish to inflict a useless service on anyone else. One of the members of the group already helped to run a day centre, and thought that they would agree to be an umbrella organisation for us, to provide help with all the paperwork involved in employing someone. She agreed to investigate that.

We decided that we had to go ahead. We could hardly back out now, although we would all have been much happier to have passed the whole model over to someone else. The day centre agreed to work with us. Now we had to have a better name. Again, we racked our brains. I rather tentatively asked if there was anyone connected with the group whose name we could use; we had been discussing fund-raising beforehand, and I wondered if we could find a donor who would like us to use their name. 'Excellent idea' came the rejoinder. 'Why don't we call it The Clive Project?' And so the second Clive in my life came into being.

We had a name. We had the offer of some money. We had the offer of help with all the legal side of taking on employees. Someone knew the friend of a friend who worked in marketing and PR, and they kindly designed a logo for us. We organised and held a very successful auction of promises which raised over £5000. Together with the money we had been promised, this made us confident we could keep going for at least the first year. Everything looked set for go. There was one small problem – we no longer had any customers. It was by now some 18 months since the original research, and younger onset dementia is in most cases a progressive illness: it can progress very fast, particularly in the absence of drugs to treat the symptoms. Clive had been living at home at the start of the research project, but was by now in a nursing home.

We held a somewhat heated argument about what to do next. A few of the group were in favour of redoing the research to identify likely clients. The rest of us wanted to go ahead and recruit some support workers, while at the same time trying to identify possible clients. We had good links through the OPTIMA project with some likely people, and I was convinced that, if we provided a genuinely helpful service, news of it would spread by word of mouth. Our research worker printed off many hundreds of Clive Project publicity leaflets, and we distributed these around anywhere we thought people with younger onset dementia, or their families, or friends, or indeed anyone with any possible interest might see them. We also decided on an open referral system. Because we received money from charitable trusts, the support we hoped to provide had to be targeted at people with younger onset dementia, but we wanted to have as few restrictions as possible. The support would be available to anyone who was under 65 at the onset of symptoms, but we wouldn't withdraw the service the day after their 65th birthday. We would hope to continue the support as long as it was useful to the person supported.

We also placed an advert in the local paper to recruit The Clive Project's first support workers, who started working for us in April 1998. We intentionally started in a fairly small way: two support workers for eight hours per week each. This was partly because of finances, but also because no-one was sure if the support would prove to be as good in practice as it seemed in theory. I wasn't involved in either the selection or the training of these two part-time workers. At the time I was seeing Clive through his first move from one home to another.

Although there were a few hiccups as support workers, people with dementia and their families started to work together, on the whole the operation was very successful, and within six months we recruited another two support workers and took on more clients. The One-to-One service has expanded steadily ever since, and is much appreciated by the users of the service and their families and friends.

The reason the support works so well is that it is entirely driven by the needs and interests of the person supported, and the support is provided, if at all possible, consistently at the same time of day by the same support worker. A relationship can develop between the support worker and the person supported, and the routine so important to the person with dementia can be maintained. The Project support team tries to match the support worker to the person with dementia, so that if possible they share interests and are likely to get on well together. Support workers are chosen for their quiet, competent, friendly attitude, and the training they receive increases that competence. We try to make contact with people who receive a diagnosis of younger onset dementia as soon as possible after diagnosis, so they can if they wish become familiar with The Project and attend some of the social events before any support is necessary. We try and provide support as soon as it is felt necessary, to maintain a good standard of living for the person with dementia, and their family and friends. By making contact at an early stage, we can take advantage of the abilities of the person with dementia to make new relationships and learn new things, before those abilities are lost as their illness progresses (if it does – not all dementias are progressive).

The Clive Project supports people who are living on their own in their own home: those who are living with their family, and those who are living in some sort of sheltered housing or care home. When an agreement has been made to provide support, a blank A4 notebook is left at the house which becomes a diary for recording visits by the support worker, and brief details of the activities involved. The diary can also be used to communicate between the family of the person with dementia and the support worker, and any other support workers who come to the house.

A typical Clive Project session starts with the support worker coming to the home of the person supported. When they arrive, the support worker will talk to the person with dementia and their partner, or look in the diary to see if a message has been left. The support worker and the person with dementia will agree on the activity for the session, which may be inside or outside. Typical activities supported are baking, gardening, playing golf, going to concerts or going for a walk. If the outing involves a car journey, that provides an good opportunity to talk about anything that may be of concern. The activity normally lasts about two and a half hours. At the end, they return home, have a cup of tea or coffee, fill in the diary and talk to the partner, and then the support worker leaves.

This structure gives a relaxed outing, time for talk, and a definite ending point so the support worker can leave without upsetting anyone. The diary is an essential means of communication between support worker, partner and any other professional carers, and also a record which the person with dementia and their partner can look back on later.

Chapter 10

The Present

It is now over nine years since Clive died. In some ways everything is different, and in other ways it is just the same.

The children, of course, have changed. They were on the verge of turning into teenagers when he died. He had been living in a nursing home for the previous two years, and they had visited progressively less often once he failed to recognise them. So the principal effect his death had on their lives was that I was around more. It also made the vexed question of family life easier to talk about at school. They gave me a reason to get out of bed in the morning, and otherwise kept me on the straight and narrow.

Now my daughter is away at college, where she is reading physics (I didn't intentionally influence her choice). My son is doing A-levels, and prefers listening to CDs and playing computer games to thinking about what he's going to do next year. They give every indication of being normal teenagers, except that one topic of conversation is forbidden in the house. They are very supportive of my work with The Clive Project and the Alzheimer's Society, but they don't want to talk about dementia, their father, or his illness. I hope the time will come when they want to know more, and I have tried to write the family anecdotes down, and sort the photographs out, so the information is available if and when they are ready. And if they are never interested, then that's OK too.

After a lot of thought, I have some clear ideas about what worked to help my own children get through Clive's illness in the way they have. I can't say if they would be helpful to other people, but it seems to me they are worth putting in writing.

1. Don't try to protect children by not telling them what is going on. The effects of dementia are not something that can be hidden. They will certainly notice odd happenings, and will create explanations if you don't give them one. Don't try and keep secrets, or have conversations they are entirely excluded from. If possible, involve a professional (nurse, doctor, community psychiatric nurse or similar). Make sure the explanations are at the level the children can understand. Give them the opportunity to talk and ask questions, but don't be upset or angry if they lose interest quickly. Your partner's illness may be the most important thing in your and your partner's life, but it may not be for your children.

2. If they are at school, inform the headteacher about the diagnosis and its likely outcome. If this can be done discreetly, so much the better. It will be easier for everyone if the diagnosis is not the subject of gossip at the school gate.

3. Try and fit a time into the family routine when the children can talk, together and individually, with the parent who does not have dementia. Don't force the conversation, but be ready to respond openly if necessary. If you really feel this is beyond you, try and offload the job onto another family member, or a close family friend, but there should always be

someone the children can approach, and that time should be a normal part of family life, not a special occasion.

4.   Don't allow the children to exploit the situation. Unless they spend a lot of time helping to care, or to run the house, having a parent with younger onset dementia is not an excuse for not getting homework done, or for getting out of games if it is raining.

5.   Don't be too gloomy about the future. There are some essential steps you need to take, mentioned in Chapter 4, but, once you have done that, try and take each day as it comes.

6.   Build treats into the routine. The diagnosis of younger onset dementia is never a laughing matter, but it is not an immediate death sentence. You may have many years of quality time to come – make the most of them.

7.   If there is any activity or holiday you have always promised yourself or your children, try and do it as early as possible.

8.   What the family needs is consistent, long-term support. I found this particularly important for my own children. There may be particular short-term issues where a brief period of counselling or intervention may help, but if long-term support is difficult (and it is for many organisations) it may be better to put the effort into supporting the adults who have most contact with the children. I certainly got a lot of support from an organisation called SeeSaw, which supports families and children who have lost a parent. I didn't always talk to the same person, but I

didn't have to start every conversation with a long preamble about who I was, and the family background.

The Clive Project has grown hugely. As well as the original researcher, who is still with the project, we now have 13 support workers supporting 48 individuals with dementia and their families and friends. Some support workers work only a few hours each week, and some work full-time; all are very much appreciated by both the people they support and the rest of us.

We made a successful bid to the Lottery for funding, and now employ two people to support the families and friends of those with younger onset dementia. The rather clumsy 'Family and Friends' terminology is the best we could manage: I was never happy with being described as Clive's 'carer', and that feeling seems quite common. It seems to diminish both the carer and the caree in the eyes of society at large. The Project has an active social calendar, with boat trips, garden parties, Christmas parties and trips to the theatre where all are welcome. We produce a newsletter three times a year. There is a very active group of family and friends, who organise talks and social gatherings, and a 'moving on' group has just started, to support those whose partner no longer lives with them.

The Project has also formed links with other organisations working with people with younger onset dementia, and has started a regional forum for groups around Oxfordshire, which meets every six months, and has now been copied in many other regions. There is even a very similar service in Worcestershire, which was set up as a copy of The Clive Project, and has been running successfully for almost a year.

There are more services available for people with younger onset dementia, but it is very much a postcode lottery. Some regions have an excellent service, some have a few services, and some regions still like to pretend that such people do not exist, or can fit into existing services. There are drugs available to help delay symptoms – they don't work for some people, and they only treat the symptoms, not the underlying cause, but I've met many people who have been given a few more years with their families and lives intact. However, now the NHS refuses to fund treatment for those in the early stages – it is not 'cost effective', though they are very unwilling to come forward and explain how they reached this conclusion. NICE talks comfortingly of them being available to people with 'moderate dementia'.[2] Clive would not have qualified until a year after he was diagnosed, by which time he was incapable of understanding most of what was said to him, and had been incapable of independent living for two or three years. And the test (the Mini-Mental State Exam) on which they base the diagnosis of 'moderate dementia' takes at most five minutes.

I think on the whole we coped with Clive's illness better than anyone could have hoped. By 'we', I mean his entire extended family, the staff at the various nursing homes, the staff at OPTIMA, but above all Clive himself.

Many of my friends were incredulous when I told them I was writing about Clive's illness. How on earth could I face reliving such times, and why should I want to? The idea came from the early days of The Clive Project, and the chance comment of one of my colleagues at work, who remarked that Clive's dementia had effects she would never have imagined. Dementia is the illness that no-one likes to think about, and most people forget if they can. People become non-people as soon as they are diagnosed. Such must have been the underlying thought of the consultant who never felt the need to tell Clive about his diagnosis, and the many people who talked to me about Clive in front of him. Clive was never prepared to put up with this; he was very open about his illness, but never thought it diminished his

2   National Institute for Health and Clinical Excellence (2006) *NICE clinical guideline 42. Dementia: supporting people with dementia and their carers in health and social care* Available at www.nice.org.uk/nicemedia/pdf/CG042NICEGuideline.pdf, accessed on 3 September 2008

rights or his personality. Alas, what it did eventually diminish was his ability to use language to communicate, and then his understanding of the world about him, but the underlying personality was always there, and visible not just to those who knew him well. The staff at the final nursing home came to Clive's funeral, and talked movingly about his sense of humour, tenacity and consideration for others. I'm sure some of that came from the reflections of Clive they saw in his family and friends, but a lot came from Clive himself. Yet when they first met Clive he had totally lost his speech, and no longer recognised his family.

The thing I am most thankful for is that we are still a family. Just after Clive was diagnosed, I wrote that I hoped that the children would remember him with affection, and still be talking to me. They do, and they are.

This book is not for Clive, because he is no longer with us. It is for all the other younger people with dementia, and their families and friends, in the hope that they can learn from his experiences, and maybe their lives can be just a little bit easier.